SHOULDERS, UPPER BACK & NECK:

Free Yourself from **PAIN!**

by:

Rosemarie Atencio

Also by Rosemarie Atencio:

Carpal Tunnel Syndrome: How to Relieve & Prevent Wrist "Burnout"!

SHOULDERS, UPPER BACK, & NECK:

Free Yourself from **PAIN!**

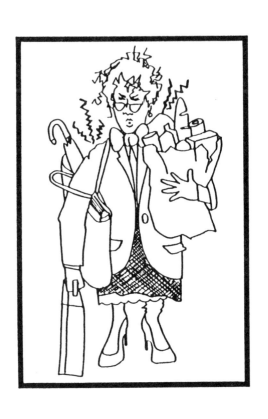

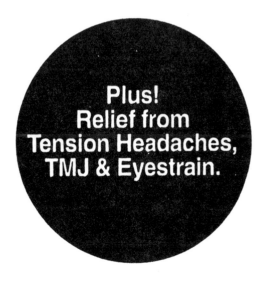

Plus!
Relief from
Tension Headaches,
TMJ & Eyestrain.

by Rosemarie Atencio

Shoulders, Upper Back & Neck
Free Yourself from **PAIN!**

Published by: **HWD Publishing**
PO Box 220
Veneta, OR 97487

Publisher's Cataloging-in-Publication Data:
Atencio, Rosemarie
Shoulders, upper back & neck: free yourself from PAIN!
/Rosemarie Atencio —- 1st ed.
p. cm.
Includes glossary and index

Defines sources of pain and strain in the upper body; provides information on self-care, exercises, postural and ergonomic changes.

1. Overuse injuries—Treatment. 2. Pain. I. Title
616.87—dc20   94-79485

ISBN #0-9637360-9-4(pbk)

This book is dedicated to Jake and Barney
and their folks.

Acknowledgements

This book came about through the help and cooperation of so many loving people whose only payment is this public thanks. Topping that special list is Dr. Sandra Ehsan who encouraged and helped me through the whole editing process. Now, that's a true friend!

My other unpaid but not unsung editors whom I would like to thank are Todd Lessner and Cristina Atencio Lessner. Also, a big thanks to Dr. Gary Blair who edited certain chapters for me in spite of his very busy practice.

To my dear friends, Jan Cox and Stan Hall, who were willing to give up their precious free time to model for the exercises. Thank you for your patience and fun attitude through the photo shoot. Additional thanks to Jan for letting me speak to the King. (I'm mentioning him in hopes that he will call again.)

To all the folks who suggested titles for the book. I would like to specially recognize Bonnie Hirsch from the Eugene Public Library. She not only submitted the first suggested title, but being a librarian, she also did the research to make sure her title was not already taken.

Special thanks to Linda Frazier for copy editing this book in the time frame that I requested. Thanks to Peter McCallum for all of the illustrations.

A big thank you to Molly Green who works so hard and is so dedicated to seeing my projects through. Also, thank you to Patsy Dunham who provided the cataloging data so promptly.

To my publisher friends, Mary Thompson and Kalyn Wolf Gibbens who share and commiserate with me, my deepest and sincere thanks for cheering me on.

ACKNOWLEDGEMENTS

Last, but certainly not least, I want to acknowledge the readers of my book on carpal tunnel syndrome who wrote to thank me and tell me how much the book has helped them. Your letters give me the incentive to continue to write books on self-care. Thank you.

Table of Contents

TABLE OF CONTENTS

TABLE OF CONTENTS

A Word from Rosemarie...

As a health practitioner and ergonomic consultant, I wrote this book because of the lack of accessible information about problems of the shoulders, upper back and neck. I found many good books on problems of the spine but they tend to focus on the lower back. This is interesting in light of the statistics that show that more than 50% of all repetitive motion injuries involve the upper body and upper extremities.

Upper body and extremities injuries are on the rise. This is to be expected because our jobs now require more upper body activity and stamina whereas our lifestyles are becoming more sedentary. The *variety* of body movements has lessened and *repetitions* have increased as we work more and more with and at machines. The long-term effects of such wear and tear are showing up on an aging work population. It is no wonder that the number of people complaining of tension headaches, neck strain, shoulder joint pain and upper back discomfort is increasing.

There is scarcely an adult who hasn't experienced at least one upper body ailment, be it tendinitis, rotator cuff tendinitis, tennis elbow, bursitis, frozen shoulder, thoracic outlet syndrome, whiplash or one of many unnamed problems. Sometimes we know the source, sometimes we do not. Sometimes we rest, avoid the activity, and get better without seeing the doctor. Sometimes we go to the doctor immediately. Usually we wait until the problem is unbearable.

Why do we wait? We wait because we are busy and muscle pain isn't considered life-threatening. We wait because we hope that the pain will just go away. We wait because we think that others might regard us as complainers.

Is there another way? Yes, there is. It is to educate yourself. With this book you will learn the way your body functions best. You do not need to study anatomy, physiology or kinesiology to learn how to take care of

A WORD FROM ROSEMARIE...

---

yourself. The rules are simple. You can restore your body to its proper functioning. You have already started by buying this book.

After you have read and applied the techniques described in this book, please let me hear from you. You can write to me in care of the publisher. I read and respond to all letters.

Stay well,

Rosemarie Atencio, HHP, LMT

REASONS

and

CAUSES

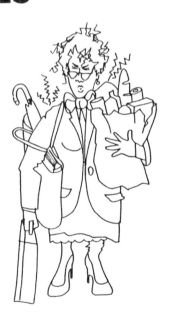

Chapter 1

Giving Grief...

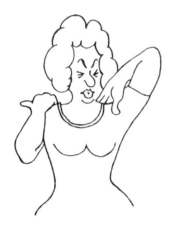

Your neck and shoulders ache. There is an aggravating twinge in your back between your shoulder blades. Your shoulder hurts every time you try to move your arm and you frequently get tension headaches. Whether you are in constant pain or the pain comes and goes, there are steps you can take to help yourself. In the following chapters, you will receive information on how to rid yourself of the source of your pain and keep the pain from coming back. You will learn:

✿ Four simple postural rules that will keep your body happy all day.

✿ Stretching and strengthening exercises for your upper body that take less than 5 minutes.

✿ Stress relieving techniques such as self-massage, artful breathing, and acupressure points.

✿ How to relieve tension headaches, eyestrain and TMJ (TMJ has to do with the jaws. It is described in subsequent chapters)

✿ How to wake up in the morning without experiencing pain in the neck and shoulders.

✿ How to make sure that you have the best pillow for your needs.

✿ Which vitamins and minerals specifically help muscles and joints.

✿ What role water plays in relieving pain and hastening healing.

Every chapter of this book explains, in easy and simple terms, how to relieve pain in your shoulders, upper back and neck. There are a *dozen*

Section I: REASONS AND CAUSES

chapters just on particular techniques you can use to help yourself. At the back of the book, there is information for specific personal treatment of tendinitis and sprains. Also, at the back of the book is a chart to help you to create your own personal plan of action.

This is your opportunity to help yourself. What could be better than living everyday without pain? Free yourself from those wear and tear injuries. Learn what you can do to help yourself avoid or relieve bursitis, frozen shoulder, rotator cuff tenditis, thoracic outlet syndrome and many other shoulder, upper back and neck disorders.

By the time you have finished reading this book, you will know the reasons and causes for pain symptoms and methods for getting relief. You will also know how to get to the source of your problem.

Every chapter in the following pages is designed to relieve your pain. Read, make notes, and apply the learning. Make the changes suggested and you will feel better immediately.

Chapter 2

The Whys and Wherefores...

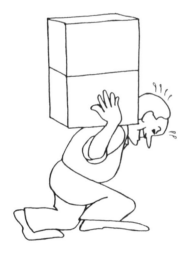

Why do I get pain in my neck and my shoulders? That is a good question to ask yourself. Let's look first at some of the commonly diagnosed disorders of the upper body and extremities. Starting with the shoulder they are: Tendinitis, bursitis, rotator cuff tendinitis, tennis elbow, golfer's elbow, frozen shoulder, carpal tunnel syndrome, thoracic outlet syndrome and ganglionic cyst. Disorders of the head and neck include: Wryneck, whiplash, stiff neck, Bell's palsy, headaches and TMJ. Let's also look at the main reason these problems occur. For the sake of clarity, I have separated the main causal factors of upper body and upper extremity disorders into four divisions. They are:

Congenital factors or chronic disease factors including muscle or nerve anomalies (something that deviates in some way from the norm), arteriosclerosis, thyroid disorders, gall bladder disorders, gout, diabetes, rheumatoid arthritis, alcoholism and gynecological disorders.

Trauma factors including accidents of all sorts such as whiplash, fractures, sprains, and lacerations.

Non-Occupational factors including athletic activities such as golf, racket sports, or baseball, and hobbies such as knitting, sewing, or gardening.

Section I: REASONS AND CAUSES

Occupational factors including poor posture, high repetitions, continuous force, inappropriate work environment or tools, improper tool use, and excessive stress.

The focus of this book is on the occupational and non-occupational problems and their solutions. Even though the information in this book may not be specific to your particular job, hobby or athletic activity, you will be able to use the information to observe and modify what you are doing.

Chapter 3

The Halves that Make a Whole...

Part of getting rid of pain in the shoulders, upper back and neck involves proper work station design and equipment. (Notice that I used the word "part".) The belief that ergonomically correct design will completely solve the problem is erroneous because it does not take the human factor into consideration.

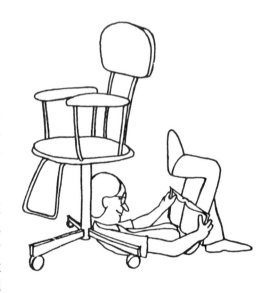

There are many well-intentioned employers who buy every ergonomic device they or the Occupational Safety and Health Agency (OSHA) can think of in order to help employees. I've had many conversations with employers who hoped that with the purchase of proper equipment, their employees would no longer experience repetitive strain injuries. Would that it were so!

 You see, ergonomically correct equipment is only half of the solution. The other half is **you**. Unless you have knowledge about the way your body functions best, you may not know how to adjust that chair, that tool, or that work station to fit your highly individual needs.

In no way do I want to indicate that ergonomically correct tools or proper work station design are not necessary. In fact, I firmly believe that correct tools are very important. What I want to make clear is that correct equipment is only part of the equation. In conjunction with the equipment,

Section I: REASONS AND CAUSES

there must also be correct tool use, appropriate posture, and other health considerations.

I have a theory on why the human factor is not fully taken into consideration. I think it is because of the emphasis on *doing* instead of *being*. In my workshops, I often ask the participants if they were all the same size when they started school at five years of age. The reply is always, "Of course not." I then ask if the tables and chairs provided took their size differences into consideration. (See previous reply.) Throughout our school years, we have adjusted ourselves to fit the desks and equipment that were provided for us. We have learned to sit quietly for longer and longer periods of time. We have learned to ignore the need of our body to move. As a result, we have developed the idea that it is up to us to adjust our bodies to the environment instead of adjusting the environment to our bodies. Along the way, we have learned to suppress our natural body wisdom in order to get the task done.

Most of us have carried the habit of ignoring our body into our adult years. When we were young, our bodies were flexible. We could break or ignore the few rules for maintaining a healthy body. We could sit on our leg without experiencing spine, hip or shoulder pain. We could lie on the floor on our tummy and read or color without low back, shoulder or neck pain. Joints, muscles, connective tissue - all of it were young and flexible.

Chapter 3: THE HALVES THAT MAKE A WHOLE...

However, as we age, the body gets cranky and it is not so agreeable about doing what we want it to do. We don't bounce back as fast as we once did. The years of thoughtless actions add up and finally - voila! - we have tightness in our upper back, our neck won't turn very far, we hurt right between the shoulder blades, or we get frequent headaches. We want to make it better but we don't know how.

Making it better includes the need to develop a sense of where our body is in the space we occupy. We need to observe ourselves in order to get back to the knowledge of our body's needs. Otherwise, all of the ergonomically correct equipment in the world will not completely solve the problem.

Recently, I saw a photo that accompanied an article which helps make the point about equipment being only part of the solution. This magazine article was about the problems of cumulative trauma injuries as they relate to musicians. Along with the article, there was a photo of the violin section of a symphony orchestra.

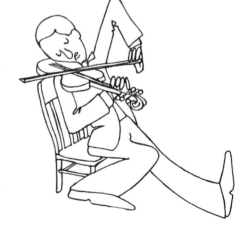

(Musicians who play stringed instruments tend to have more overuse or misuse disorders than other musicians.) What I noticed about the photo was the difference in the way that two of the violinists were holding their violins and bows. Even though the violinists were using the same instrument, their wrist and arm positions were quite different. One violinist was sitting up straight with his bow in perfect alignment. The other violinist was holding his bow at an awkward angle making him a likely candidate for serious problems in the future. Not only that, he was slouching in his chair in a way that placed his hips and shoulders at an angle that forced his back into an exaggerated curve. He did not seem to know what his body was doing in the space that he occupied. It was obvious that no one had taught him the rules of good body mechanics.

It is important to be conscious of what you are doing and how you are doing it. After all, even though muscle and tendon misuse and overuse may not be life-threatening, the quality of life suffers greatly from such problems. A good quality of life requires full range of motion, maximum flexibility and avoidance of chronic muscle and joint problems.

Keep in mind that **you** are at least half of the ergonomic equation. To get to know that half better, we will devote the rest of this section of the book to learning about the relationships of the upper body and extremities. This is a wonderful opportunity to find out just how fantastic you are.

Chapter 4

Relationships to Last a Lifetime...

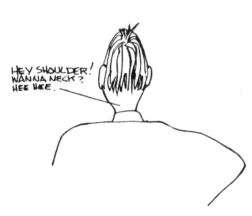

What magnificently complex structures and relationships make up your shoulders, upper back and neck! The type of joints and the way muscles connect to the joint create the range of motion that is available to you. A basic knowledge of how the joints and muscles work is necessary for you to understand the importance of your posture and actions. (Whenever I use the word muscles, I am referring to the muscles and their tendons. It is actually the tendon of the muscle that attaches to the joints.)

Basically, there are two determinates of movement and position; they are the joints and muscles. The type of joint (your body has six different types) determines the range of joint movement. For example, the ball and socket joint of the shoulder/arm provides you with a large *potential* range of movement. By comparison, the hinge joint of the elbow provides a limited *possibility* for motion.

The only way your joint can actually move is when muscles move it. The words "potential" and "possibility" in the last paragraph refer to the relationship of muscle to muscle and muscle to joint. It takes precise cooperation between muscle and joint to hold you erect and provide you with action. (Ligaments attach bone to bone and also help to stabilize the joints and keep your joint erect.) Whenever any one of these relationships is out of synchronization, you experience limited movement, achiness, or referred pain. (Referred pain means that pain is experienced in one area but the source is in another area.)

Section I: REASONS AND CAUSES

To understand how the joints and muscles operate together, roll your head down so that your chin is resting on your chest. Feel the pull down your back as the muscles are stretched and the joints of the spine bow outward. You have called into use many muscles. These muscles are tugging on bones in order to provide movement. (There are muscles that extend down from the base of your skull to the middle of your spine. This is why pain in the upper back often refers pain to the neck and shoulders and vice versa.)

One of the major relationships of joint and muscle is at the shoulder and arm. As I mentioned earlier, this ball and socket type joint has the most extensive range of movements of any joint in your body. (Due to the great range of movement that is available, it is also one of the easiest joints to dislocate.) Muscles and ligaments come from all directions to provide support and movement to this joint. All of the muscles are expanding and contracting as necessary to move the joint anyway you request, up to the limits of the joint.

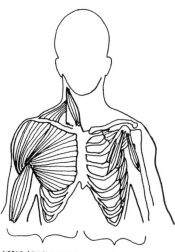

UPPER MUSCLE LAYER   LOWER MUSCLE LAYER
MUSCLES: SHOULDER, NECK & CHEST

Relating to and equally important to the movement of the shoulder/arm joint is the pectoralis or "pec" muscles. The pecs make up most of the muscles of the chest. To experience the relationship of the pec muscles to the shoulders, stretch your shoulders back and notice how pulling the arms back stretches the pecs. Now, move in the opposite direction and feel the pecs pulling on your shoulders. Most of our work nowadays stretches the back and contracts the pecs. In a subsequent chapter, this "push-me, pull-me" relationship and its connection to upper back and shoulder pain will be discussed more fully.

Chapter 4: RELATIONSHIPS TO LAST A LIFETIME...

The junction between shoulder and neck also share a bone and muscle relationship. It is a rare event when someone has pain in the neck and no pain in the shoulders or the reverse. That is because many of the same muscles that serve the shoulders also serve the neck. For example, try raising your shoulders. The muscles that just raised your shoulders are attached both at the shoulder wings and at the base of your skull. In that way, when you contract or pull the muscles

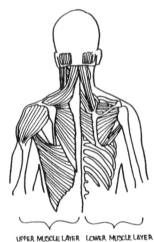

UPPER MUSCLE LAYER LOWER MUSCLE LAYER
MUSCLES: SHOULDER, NECK & BACK

to raise your shoulder, you are bringing the shoulder closer to the neck. (Quite a few of the upper back and shoulder muscles terminate at the base of the skull. That is why tension headaches often start in that area.)

The complex relationship of all of the muscles and joints, how they attach and where they attach make it difficult to pinpoint the source of pain and discomfort. In this book, there is information on correct posture and exercises to help relieve or prevent pain in the muscles and joints of the shoulders, upper back and neck.

Healthy muscles and joints are essential for pain-free movement, but they are not the only components in the entire picture. In the next chapter, you will get to know three other important players.

Chapter 5

Those Three Little Words...

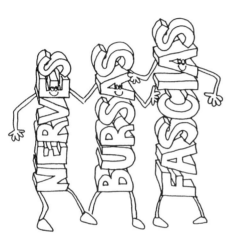

Three important contributors to movement in your shoulders, upper back and neck are the nerves, bursas and fascias (fash-ee-ahs.) Problems diagnosed as bursitis, thoracic outlet syndrome, and myofascial trigger points are all ways of describing some sort of limitation or pain in movement in which nerve, bursa or fascia are involved. For ease of explanation, I will describe the role of each component separately.

The first component we will look at is the nerves. Once the decision to move is made, the nerves carry the messages to and from the muscles. The process may sound slow and ponderous but actually nerve impulses travel at a <u>minimum</u> of 135 miles per hour!

All nerves exit the spinal column and go branching and coursing throughout the body. Pictures of nerves leaving the spine look like a tree with limbs, branches and twigs. If you've ever laid in the grass staring up into a tree, then you know what the spine and nerve branches look like. Three of the main nerve branches leave the spine at the neck, dive under the collarbone, and continue their journey to the hands and fingers. These particular nerves are involved in the motor and sensory actions of the neck, shoulders, arms, hands and fingers. These nerves can be caught or pinched by inflamed muscles or between bones and muscles. The unhappy nerve can refer pain sensations anywhere along the pathway from the neck all the way down to the fingers. This is what makes the diagnosis of carpal tunnel syndrome a little tricky. Since the sensations you are experiencing in the hand and fingers may actually originate in the shoulders or neck. (However, if the sensations are found to be carpal tunnel syndrome, please refer to my book, <u>Carpal Tunnel Syndrome: How to Relieve & Prevent Wrist "Burnout"!</u>)

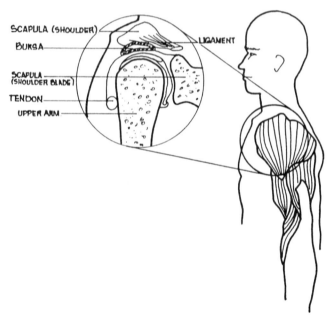

The second component you need to know about is the bursa. Almost everyone has heard of "bursitis." People leave the doctor's office reciting, "The doctor said I have bursitis." But, what does that mean? "Itis" means inflammation. Therefore, you have inflammation of a bursa. And what is a bursa? It's a sac of fluid that keeps the joint lubricated and keeps the tendons from rubbing on the bone. We have lots of these little lubricating stations in our bodies. The one in your shoulder is often blamed for shoulder pain.

The last component, which is not as well known as the nerve or bursa, is the fascia. This fascinating material is everywhere in your body. It is commonly called connective tissue and it consists mostly of collagen. Your tendons, ligaments, and bones are made of it. It completely outlines your body just as the skin does and it lies just below the skin holding up your innards. It separates and protects organs, it acts as a sheath for nerves, muscles, and blood vessels, and it encases the brain and spinal cord. Fascia is so strong that it takes about 2,000 pounds per square inch of force to rip it!

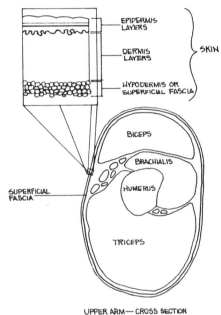

Another way to explain fascia is to recall the process of removing the skin from a chicken. You probably noticed that as you lifted the skin away from the body there was a tough somewhat opaque layer between the skin and the muscle that made it difficult to pull the skin off. That is fascia.

Unlike bone and muscle, connective tissue or fascia does not have a rich blood supply. Since blood is the river that carries the healing nutrients, a sprain or strain can take a long time to heal, and a tendon can require much patience and care before it is completely healed.

UPPER ARM—CROSS SECTION

Now that you have followed the explanations of the separate components, let's look at how they act together. Muscles receive messages from the nerves and either contract or expand according to the messages. This, in turn, causes the tendon to pull on the bone and you have movement. Lubricating stations (bursas) keep the tendons separated and lubed as the tendons move. Ligaments provide stability to the joint. All the while, fascias are providing separation, protection, stability and encasement to the muscles and joints. Notice that everything has to coordinate for movement. Head to neck, neck to shoulder, shoulder to arm and arm to hand. In order to do that, some muscles have to relax and be stretched while other muscles are contracted and working. This cooperation of muscles is the subject of the next chapter.

Chapter 6

Push Me, Pull Me

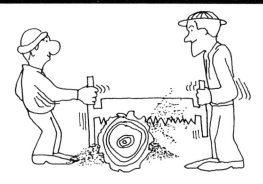

Muscles need to cooperate with each other for movement. In other words, every group of muscles must be in balance with its opposing muscle group in order to generate maximum action. This muscle balance and cooperation can be likened to two men on a cross-cut saw - one pushing and expanding while the other is simultaneously pulling and contracting.

A good example of balanced and opposing muscle groups is the biceps and triceps which are located in front and back, respectively, of the upper arm. If you want to bring your hand closer to your shoulder, a cooperative effort between these two muscle groups is needed - the biceps need to shorten or contract and the triceps need to lengthen or expand. All muscles need and rely on this mutual cooperation to function properly.

The muscles of the neck also provide a good example of the need for balanced activity. One side of the neck has muscles of the same shape, size, and action potential as the other side. If you want to bring your ear closer to your shoulder on one side, not only does that side need to contract, but also the other side needs to expand or lengthen as well.

Referring back to the two men on a cross-cut saw, what if one man could not cooperate? Under those circumstances, no

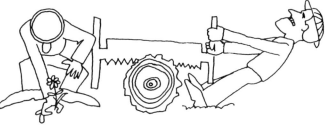

movement could take place. This is an important aspect of balance and cooperation in muscles. If, for example, one side of the neck is tense or has spasms in it, motion becomes limited or impossible. The balance and cooperation between each side has been lost. If the limited movement is not corrected, the neck will have less and less range of movement. (Very often the tension or spasm in a muscle is caused by incorrect posture. Postural problems can be brought about by the tools we use, the way we use them, the environment in which we work or play, the sleep positions we maintain and the amount of rest and recuperation we get.)

Interestingly, tension and spasm in a muscle are more likely to occur from holding an expanded or lengthened position for too long than from being shortened or contracted. An example that almost everyone has experienced is using the neck to cradle the phone while talking. The side of the neck that has been stretched experiences pain and limitation. Think about what this means. Almost all of our activities involve forward motion for example, driving a car, working at a computer, or doing assembly work. In these posi- 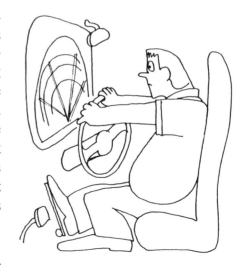 tions, the upper back and shoulders are straining forward. It's no wonder that the area between the shoulder blades feels tight and painful. Balance and cooperation need to be maintained between the back and front (pec) muscles.

Section 1: REASONS AND CAUSES

In the example of forward work, the upper back and shoulders will feel tense and maybe even painful. What needs to happen to maintain balance is that the shoulders need a break from lengthening. That break can take the form of stretch - but not of the back. The back has already been stretched. The muscles that need stretching are the pecs which have been contracted or shortened. In this way, the shoulders, upper back and neck will have a chance to relax. If the balance between opposite muscles is not maintained, the muscles develop chronic spasms and pull on the bones to which they are attached until the posture is affected.

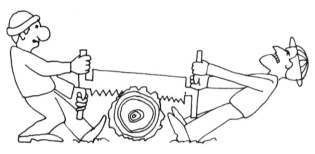

Again, using the two men on a cross-cut saw to describe an action, what would happen if one man was strong and the other man was weak? How long could the strong man compensate for the weak one? In time, the strong man would be exhausted and overworked. The same thing happens when one muscle or group of muscles is injured or in pain and other muscles try to compensate. That is why it is so important to respond to pain and discomfort in the early stages. The longer that compensation continues, the more muscles become involved. Eventually, the entire shoulder, upper back or neck hurts and it can take a long time for the problem to be reversed. It is not possible to put too much emphasis on the need to act when problems first arise.

Chapter 7
The Shoulder Bone's Connected to the Neck Bone...

Do you remember that old song about how the bones are all connected? Well, the same thing could be said about muscles. No movement, no action, and no pose takes place in a vacuum. Every move and every posture is an interactive event. Something is affecting something else.

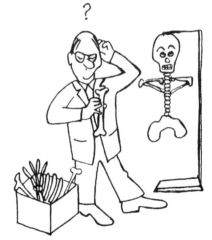

Have you ever rubbed somebody's back and noticed that some of the muscles felt as taut as a stretched out rope or as rigid as a tabletop? Muscles that have been in a chronic (long time) state of ropiness or rigidity can be very difficult to convince to let go and relax.

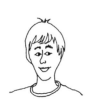

There are many theories as to why muscles remain so stubbornly hard, but an explanation of them wouldn't bring us any closer to understanding the ways to prevent pain. *Instead, it is important to remember that holding a position for a long time or doing the same movement over and over again breaks the basic rules for maintaining strong, healthy muscles and bones.*

As an example, imagine someone doing forward work all day. This means that they are stretching the upper back and shoulders while contracting the pecs. Remembering that a muscle's tendon attaches to the bone and pulls the bones to provide movement. What do you think is happening to the bones of the shoulder in this case? If you said they would be pulled out of alignment, you are correct.

Try the position. Can you feel the pull across the back and the contraction of the pecs? Can you imagine what would happen to you if you maintained that position throughout the day - day after day? In time, you would become "round-shouldered." However, that is not all of it. There is even more happening to the bones and muscles.

What do you suppose is happening to your spine? Try the position again. Can you feel the pull across the spine? Add a little slouch by dropping your ribs into your hips. Notice the increased strain across the upper back and the bowing of the spine. This is known as "khyphosis" (ki-fo-sis). Tendons that reach from the spine to the arms, shoulders and neck pull on the spine. Not only does this action bow the spine, but it also causes the muscles to remain in a chronic state of stretching. This explains some of the rigidity in the muscles we discussed at the beginning of the chapter, but wait... there's more...

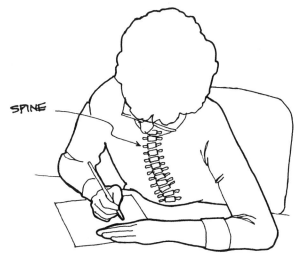

SPINE

As I mentioned in the title of this chapter, everything is connected, so what about the neck? As you slouch and place your arms and shoulders forward, what is happening to your neck? In a slouched position, your neck is bowing forward, your chin is coming up, and your head is dropping back. This bowing forward of the neck is known as "lordosis" which is the opposite of khyphosis. Not only does this strain the muscles, tendons and ligaments, but the pressure on spinal discs can lead to problems along the nerve pathways. You might not feel pain at the neck, but you might be waking up at night with tingling, numbness or burning sensation in your fingers or hands. That

Chapter 7: THE SHOULDER BONE'S CONNECTED TO THE NECK BONE...

may make you think that it is carpal tunnel syndrome when, in fact, the problem is in the neck.

The spine naturally and gracefully undulates in and out. However, the additional and exaggerated inward and outward bowing puts a great strain on the spine and the surrounding muscles, and by the end of the day, the entire upper back and neck ache.

Let's look at another example of how this connectedness works. If the arm on your chair is too low, you compensate by resting your forearm and elbow on one arm of the chair. Try assuming the position so that you can study how it feels. Now, let's use x-ray vision and see what is going on inside.

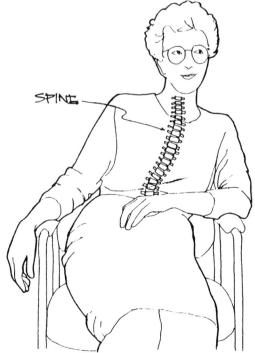

With x-ray vision, you would see that the shoulders are at an angle. The shoulder on the chair arm side would be lower and the other shoulder would be higher in order to balance the body. The force would be carried by the elbow and shoulder on the lower side - the side "resting" on the arm of the chair. (Asking a muscle to hold a load without moving is known as "static loading".) Your x-ray eyes would also notice that the neck pulls away from the resting shoulder and you would see the spine forming an "S" curve or a "scoliotic" (sko-lee-aut-ik) curve.

Section I: REASONS AND CAUSES

 In this position, not only are the bones being pulled into straining positions, but the same thing is happening to the muscles, tendons and ligaments. In the next chapter, we will look at more positions and types of movement that present problems for the upper body. See if you can identify yourself in some of these movements.

Chapter 8

The Mechanics of It All...

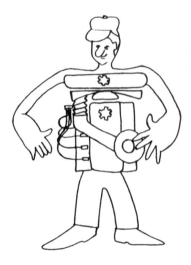

There are certain movements that create or irritate arm, shoulder, upper back and neck problems. While all of the movements we will be discussing in this chapter are within the range of motion for the body, <u>some movements put the body at a mechanical disadvantage.</u>

Let's consider an activity that the body likes best and can maintain for long periods of time without discomfort or residual problems. The activity that I am describing is walking. Think about the ease with which the shoulders and arms swing forward and back. Think of how the spine is erect with the neck easily supporting the head. Think of the lack of pain in the hands and fingers. A healthy body can do this for hours without feeling any discomfort. This position would therefore be considered the "neutral position."

The more that any part of the body is asked to deviate from this neutral position, the more stress the body experiences. Stress is increased by long hours holding the same position, high repetitions of stressful movements, and an excessive use of force or vibration. When any one or a combination of these stressors occur, the muscles, tendons, ligaments, and joints become weakened over time and develop problems.Continuous overuse or misuse leads to tendinitis, thoracic outlet syndrome, and tennis elbow - to name some of the more common ailments.

Let's look at some of the deviations from the neutral position. These deviations cause strain, inflammation or injury when repeated frequently. Let's look at some of the ways that they occur.

Section I: REASONS AND CAUSES

Shoulder/Arm:

Reaching above the shoulder

This movement can be the culprit in frozen shoulder, tendinitis, rotator cuff problems and thoracic outlet syndrome. Some examples of this motion are cutting hair with the customer's chair too high or re-stocking shelves in a library or grocery store without using a step stool or lifting heavy objects over head.

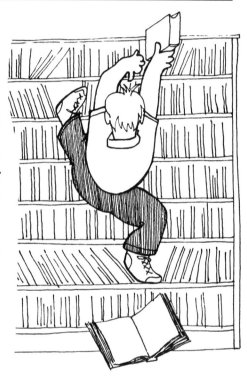

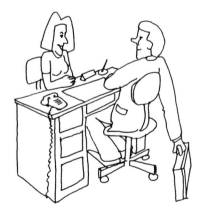

Reaching behind the body

This motion can strain the shoulders, upper arm, and chest muscles. It can also cause problems in the shoulder/arm joint. Examples of the movement include reaching behind for a book or a file instead of turning around and picking it up.

Reaching across the front and to the opposite side

This movement puts the arm and shoulder joint at maximum range, thereby, straining the joints and the arm, shoulder and back muscles. If force is added to the repetitions by lifting or hitting, then shoulder dislocation can occur. Examples of this motion can be observed in assembly work when the items are not placed conveniently. This is also seen with the backhand stroke of tennis.

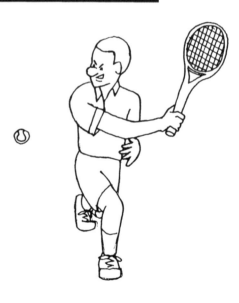

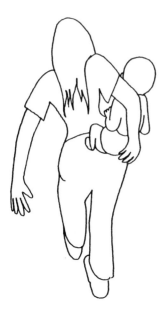

Maintaining one shoulder higher/lower than the other

This unbalanced movement not only puts undue strain on the shoulder, but often the neck and upper back are involved in an effort to offset this lopsided action. Some examples in which a shoulder can be held high include carrying a heavy shoulder bag suspended from the shoulder or using the shoulder to hold a phone. Examples of a shoulder being lower are: carrying an object on one hip or carrying a heavy parcel with one hand.

Section I: REASONS AND CAUSES

Pulling shoulders down and back

This motion strains the neck and shoulders. One of the best known examples of this action is the military stance. Another example is carrying or pulling a heavy object with the arms in back of the body.

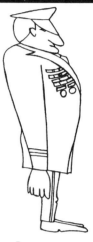

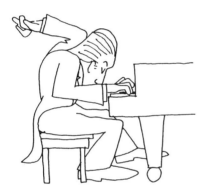

Pushing shoulders forward

This movement not only pulls on the spine, but it usually causes the head to strain forward thereby, putting stress on the neck. Examples include hunching over a desk, a table, a musical instrument or a drafting board.

Rotating the forearm when the wrist is bent

This movement puts the wrist and forearm in a position of strain that affects the forearm muscles, tendons and ligaments. Examples of this action are: using the fingers with force to hold an object while scanning or demagnetizing it or while strumming or plucking a musical instrument.

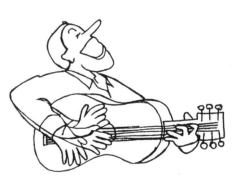

Keeping arm extended and elbow straight
This motion forces the joints and tissues to their maximum range; thereby putting them under stress. This movement can be observed when a computer mouse is used incorrectly or when lifting objects at a distance from the body.

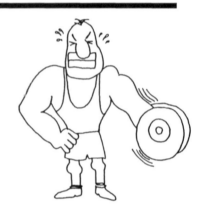

Resting weight on the elbow
This movement causes a static load on the shoulders and elbow putting the muscles under a great amount of stress. It also causes pinching of the "crazy bone" nerve which can lead to tingling or numbness in the little finger and the ring finger. This movement is noticeable when the arms of a chair are too low or when writing or drawing on a flattop surface.

Having elbow elevated or acutely bent
This movement takes the joint to its maximum range. If held for long periods of time or repeated frequently, strain on the joint and muscle can occur. Packing boxes or bags on a high surface is an example of the need to continuously elevate the elbow. Elbows are often acutely bent while holding the phone in one hand and writing with the other.

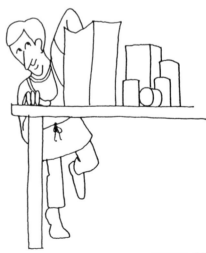

Head and Neck:

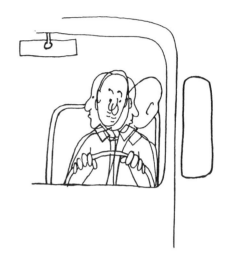

Turning head and neck

This motion is within the range of the neck but, high repetitions can bring about pain, discomfort and strain. A couple of good examples of this are seen when driving a vehicle or transcribing a document by using a computer or type-writer.

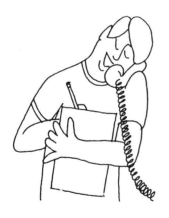

Maintaining head tilted to one side

This movement forces the body to bend towards the low area which, in turn, forces the neck to compensate by leaning more to the other side. Common examples of head tilting are: resting the phone receiver between the shoulder and neck or resting an arm on the arm of a chair that is too low. (Sleeping face up on a pillow that allows the head to pull to one side puts strain on the neck muscles even though the body isn't compensating.)

Chapter 8: THE MECHANICS OF IT ALL...

Keeping head bent forward

This motion can strain the muscles of the neck and back and lead to headaches, neck pains and upper back tightness. Examples of situations that can cause this problem are: continuous use of a microscope or a computer screen, faulty vision, ill-fitting glasses, poor posture or an inadequate work station.

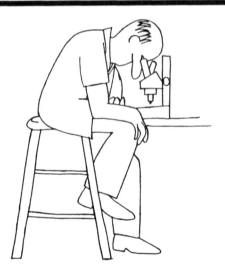

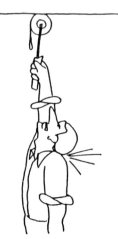

Keeping head bent back

This movement puts a great deal of strain on the front of the neck. (It can also means that the arms are working above the shoulders which brings us back to the first problem in this chapter.) Examples include painting a ceiling, working in a pit under a vehicle, or reading while lying on your stomach.

As you read through the list above, were you able to identify areas where you could improve your movements or environment? This chapter is about self-care. Start noticing everything. Notice your posture in the car, your job, home, hobbies and sports activities. Small changes can lead to big improvements.

RELIEF

and

PREVENTION

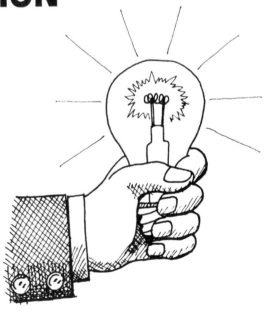

Chapter 9
I Don't Want To And You Can't Make Me

Whenever you decide to make a change that affects your body, it is a good idea to have a chat with your physical self . The body tends to lag behind a little in accepting new ideas. Have you ever noticed how your body responds when you hurl it into an exercise program? You get a notion: "we" (referring to you and your body) are going to start exercising. You go to the gym and vigorously workout. The next day, your body balks at the slightest movement.

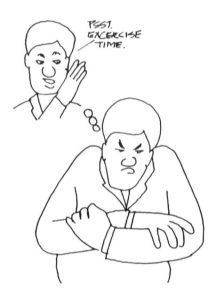

 The body responds more willingly to loving guidance than to sudden and unexpected change. Treat the body as you would a child who you are coaxing into change. It took a long time to get to your present state. Be patient and allow your body a little time to adjust to change.

Change doesn't feel right. It feels awkward. It can even be tiring. Muscles that are not use to holding you erect balk after a few minutes. Arms that haven't stretched much don't really want to do it. You need to be patient and kind with the physical part of yourself.

A good example of the need to bring the body into slow acceptance involves an employee of a local company. This employee worked for a company that takes pride in providing well for its employees. The company had just purchased expensive, ergonomically correct chairs for everyone. Within a day of receiving the new chair, this employee phoned

Section II: Relief and Prevention

me and said she was ready to throw it out. She knew I did ergonomic consulting and wanted to know what she should do. I asked her if she had gotten rid of her old chair. Fortunately, she hadn't. I suggested that first she make sure that the new chair was properly adjusted to her body. Then I suggested she try sitting and working in the new chair for about an hour. After an hour, she should return to her old chair. I also suggested that she gradually increase the time that she spends in the new chair. This will give her body a chance to get use to a new way of sitting and holding a position. I told her that the muscles and bones need time to catch up with the new concept. She called me sometime later and told me that it was well worth the extra time and patience. Now, she loves her new chair and her body is completely happy and adjusted.

It is important to remember that the physical does not operate solely at the whimsy or directives of the mental. **Think of your body as your partner instead of a slave to a mental master.**

Try to introduce change in a way that the body can slowly adapt and agree to do. Otherwise, you may be inclined to give up before you've given yourself a chance to succeed.

The chapters that follow are all about making changes so that you can enjoy freedom from pain in the neck, shoulders and upper back. Try to be patient and not let your enthusiasm for change cause you to defeat yourself. As you read these subsequent chapters, remember that you need to go slowly and be patient. Introduce change gradually and keep adding change a little at a time. In that way, your body can be your fully cooperating partner.

Chapter 10

Positioning Yourself...

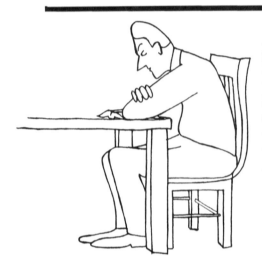

As I mentioned earlier, the body does have positions in which it operates best. Let's go over four of the basic rules of posture. Keep in mind that change comes slowly. Even though I am saying that these positions are best for the body, remember that your particular body may not be use to them. Give these changes some time to take effect and be patient with yourself.

Four Postural Rules for the Body:

1. Spine straight all the way up to the neck - no continuous turning, bending or tilting of the head.

Suggestions:

⇒ ❑ Adjust the mirrors on your vehicle while keeping your head straight and aligned over your neck. Looking through the mirrors while driving should be done with the eyes moving - not the head.

⇒ ❑ At a computer, place the screen directly in front of you - not over to one side. Use a document holder which is placed even with and right next to the screen. Make sure the top of the screen is level with your eyes and that only your eyes (not your head) need to move to see the screen or the document holder.

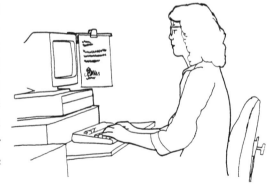

Section II: RELIEF AND PREVENTION

⇒ ❏   Prop up reading material or use a stand to avoid bending your head forward while reading. Never read while lying on your side or tummy.

⇒ ❏   Buy a writing stand or a desktop that tilts toward you and brings work closer. (Bring your desk or tabletop work to you instead of you to the work.)

⇒ ❏   If you are on the phone a lot, invest in a headset or move the phone every few minutes from one ear to the other.

⇒ ❏   Have your hearing checked. Partial deafness may be causing you to turn your head to one side in order to hear.

⇒ ❏   Make sure that you are not compensating for poorly fitted bifocals or eyeglass frames that interfere with proper vision.

⇒ ❏   Your pillow or any other surface that you use for resting your head needs to be firm and high/low enough so that your head is not tilted in either direction when you lie on your side. (Couch potato alert: You need to watch those sofa arms.)

⇒ ❏   Make sure your chair swivels if you have a work station that requires you to talk to someone behind you. (I worked with a receptionist whose neck pains ended when I suggested that she turn her entire body around instead of just her head to talk to the people behind her.)

⇒ ❏   Light needs to be directed on the object or task that you have in focus so that you won't be straining forward to see what you're doing.

2. Shoulders need to be held even, relaxed, and squared with hips.

Suggestions:

⇒ ❑ Notice if you are sitting at a angle... in the car, at your work station, or in your favorite chair. Check to see if this is because the arm of the chair is too low.

⇒ ❑ When standing, instead of placing your weight on one hip, stand with your feet about shoulder-width apart, relax your knees and distribute your weight evenly over the balls of your feet.

⇒ ❑ When you carry something, hold it in front of you, close to the body with your elbows at a right angle instead of carrying the weight on your hips.

⇒ ❑ Sit with feet on the floor rather than with legs crossed or with your leg tucked under you. If you need to cross your legs, do so only at the ankles.

⇒ ❑ Sit on your "sitting bones." (Those 2 bony projections just above the back of your thighs.) This will take tremendous pressure and strain off of your neck and shoulders. If you find that you have trouble sitting this way, it may be because one hip is higher than the other. You can tell because one sitting bone will feel like it is carrying a lot more pressure than the other. Try placing a foam wedge or small

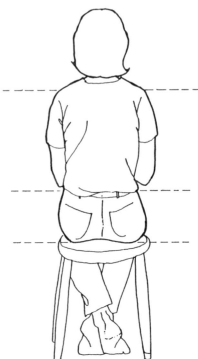

pillow under the higher side.

⇒ ❑ Avoid carrying weight on one shoulder or dragging your shoulder down by carrying weight with one hand. Either carry something that is weighty with both hands or find a carrier with wheels. If nothing else, at least shift the load to the other hip from time to time.

⇒ ❑ If you walk with a cane, notice if you carry your shoulder high on one side.

3. Arms function best when kept below and in front of the shoulder and bent 90 degrees at the elbow.

Suggestions:

⇒ ❑ Adjust the steering wheel and seat to avoid a straight-arm reach when driving.

⇒ ❑ Instead of continuously throwing heavy material such as logs or cement sacks put them in a cart and wheel the cart to the stack or pile.

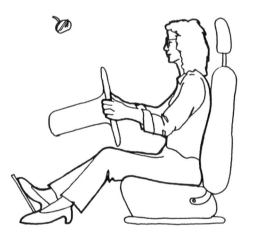

⇒ ❑ Use boxes with handles instead of wrapping your arms around the boxes.

⇒ ❑ Bring items up to counter level rather than continuously reaching down and picking the items up.

⇒ ❑ When working on fine or intricate work overhead, stand on a platform to get closer to the work. With larger areas such as a ceiling, use handle extensions to reach and stand well back from area. Stop often and look down.

⇒ ❑ Place your work directly in front of you. If you do need to reach back to get something, remember to turn completely around.

⇒ ❑ *Gradually* develop strength and flexibility in your arms and shoulders if you want to play racket sports, golf, swimming or other athletic activities that take the arm outside of the best natural range.

4. Upper back needs to be straight and aligned up and down and side to side with lower back and neck. (Here again, the upper back is pulled out of kilter when either one of the shoulders or one of the hips is higher than the other. Many of the same situations that cause imbalances in the shoulders and hips affect the upper back, too.)

Suggestions:

⇒ ❑ Slouching bows the back. (Some of my clients have learned to recite, "Get my ribs out of my hips" as a means of remembering to stop slouching.) Avoid the opposite extreme of forcing the upper body into a rigid and tense position. Instead, maintain a relaxed but upright position. (Note: Avoid sitting for long periods of time on overstuffed couches and chairs.)

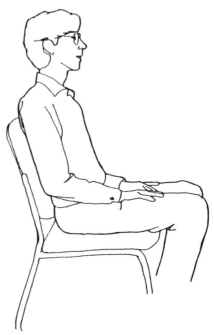

Section II: RELIEF AND PREVENTION

⇒ ❏   Watch for the tendency to hunch the shoulders forward, such as when writing at a desk that is too low for you.

⇒ ❏   Leaning into your work or reaching continuously in front of you will strain the upper back. Leaning in can be caused by inadequate eyewear. Have someone measure the distance between your work surface or computer screen and your eyes. Then have your eye doctor make up prescription glasses for that distance. Keep those particular glasses at the work area for handy use.

These are the four postural rules. Some of the rules overlap because, as I mentioned before, all parts of the body are interconnected.

Now that you've read the rules, go back over them and think of the rules in terms of what you are doing right now. Then think about the rules in terms of your daily activities. Put a checkmark in the box for those areas that you need to change. You'd be surprised how a few small changes can make all the difference in how you feel.

Remember to take the time to analyze not only what you are doing but how you are doing it. When you begin to feel achy, ask yourself, "How could I do this differently?" Whatever you do, don't just try to "plow through it."

Chapter 11

Taking Time for R & R...

When someone takes an R & R in the military, that means they are resting and recreating or resting and recuperating. In other words, they are taking a vacation or a rest from their duties. In this chapter, the R & R will stand for rest and recuperation. These two words 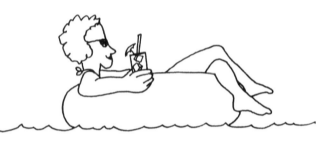 definitely belong in your health vocabulary if you want to avoid or relieve the pain and strain in the neck, shoulders and upper back.

You need rest from holding the same static position or from high repetitions of the same motion. In other words, it doesn't really matter whether you are passive or active. Whichever it is, **the body needs a change of movement - a chance to hold a different position or move in a different way.**

One of the best examples of the body's need for positional changes occurs when you are sleeping. Even though you are at rest, your body is moving and changing positions. Photographs taken while someone is asleep show that the body moves every 15-20 minutes and completely changes positions 7-8 times during the night. Why is it that the resting body continues to move and alter itself?

Let's look at the question another way... what would happen if the body didn't move during the entire night? We would be very stiff and sore in the morning. Yet we ask our body to hold sitting, standing and resting positions for long periods of time. No wonder we ache when we try to get up after sitting through a long plane flight or car ride. No wonder we feel the pull on our back when we try to sit down after

Section II: RELIEF & PREVENTION

standing for a long time. No wonder we have pain across our upper back and neck when we have been working at a computer for hours. Rest is needed from holding these positions for so long. Rest is also needed from the opposite extreme - highly repetitive motion.

The problem in the case of repetitive motion is that the same movements are repeated over and over again without the needed rests. Known by such names as cumulative trauma disorders, repetitive motion injuries, or repetitive motion strain, these repetitive motions take a toll on the body. These are wear and tear injuries where ligaments that are holding joints can destabilize, tendons holding muscles to bone can become frayed, and the voluntary muscles can become chronically inflamed. Repetitive motion is also behind such problems as scar tissue, adhesions, nerve impingement, edema and a whole host of other disorders.

The results of chronic wear and tear are the same as a sudden and traumatic injury. The difference is that repetitive motion injuries sneak up on you. **The need for an early response is essential. Don't overlook yourself.** Don't dismiss early signs of injury. Don't assume that a recurring shoulder, neck or upper back pain will continue to go away. Take action. The sooner you take care of the problem, the less likely you will be to need drugs or surgery.

In my book on carpal tunnel syndrome, I refer to "mini-vacations." These are small rests, task variations, a moment of stretching, or other small breaks taken every 15-20 minutes to give the body a rest from repetitive movement. These mini-vacations take away some of the stress that the body is feeling in doing the same movement over and over again.

Now for the other half of the "R..." Webster's Dictionary defines recuperation as "to recover health or strength." Recuperation is also the time it takes to repair ourselves.

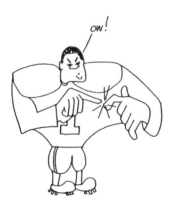

The concept of recuperation reminds me of a workshop that I conducted. The workshop was attended by workers and competitive athletes. To make a point about recuperation to the workers, I asked the athletes if they would workout in the same way 5 days a week for 8 hours a day. As I expected, the athletes collectively answered, "No way." What was there about doing the same workout everyday that they knew would not help their competitive edge? They knew that muscles need time to recuperate or recover. They knew that preventing injuries required a commitment to letting their bodies recuperate.

If what you do at work involves using the same muscles that you use for your hobbies or athletic activities, what chance does your body have to recuperate? If you are sitting all day on the job, sitting in your car driving home and then sitting all evening at home, what chance does the spine have to get relief from the pressure of sitting? If you are using a keyboard all day and spend your evenings working or 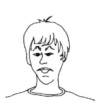 playing at a computer, when do your forearms, neck, and shoulders rest? A night's sleep may not be sufficient to help your body rebuild the wear and tear that occurs from repetitive activity day after day.

Section II: RELIEF & PREVENTION

Muscles, bones, tendons and ligaments all need time to regenerate. Even people who run or power walk regularly are advised to do so every other day and to do upper body workouts on the opposite days. These variations in routine are to allow the body to make cellular repairs and replacement.

You are a dynamic being. By that I mean that you are changing all the time. Beyond your genetic gifts, **you are a product of the actions that you take, the food that you eat, and the stress that you bring to bear on your entire self.**

Vary your activities. Notice the movements that you do all the time. Think of other things that you could do to break up the monotony and stress that the same daily actions are putting on your body.

In other chapters, there are stretches and strengthening ideas to help you in taking your R & R. Incorporate them into your habits. You will feel better, have less stress, and enjoy life more.

Chapter 12

Grandma Knew Best

When I was a little girl, my grandmother would watch me stretch and say, "Stretch and grow big." My grandmother's words were always the same and always encouraged me to stretch. Grandmother was right - I did grow bigger. OK. I know that would have happened anyway. The point is that her attention and encouragement gave me a lifelong enjoyment of stretching. I stretch all during the day.

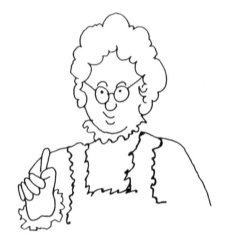

You need to stretch. Stretching is not the same as exercising. Stretching fulfills a different purpose. It is a needed respite when you have been holding a contraction (or shortening) of your muscles, tendons, fascia and ligaments for a long period. It also increases your flexibility. (Flexibility becomes important to us as we get older. The more freedom of movement we have, the more actions we can undertake without sustaining injury.)

I said that stretching is not the same as exercising. A workout done once a day is fine to meet the needs of the cardiovascular system and to build stamina. However, ten minutes of stretching done once a day won't really fill the bill for muscles and joints. Stretching is an activity that needs to be done as part of your everyday activities. Don't wait until you feel tension. **Think of stretching not so much as exercise but, like eating or satisfying thirst, something you do during the normal course of a day - all during the day.**

Section II: RELIEF AND PREVENTION

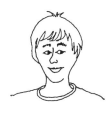

You can start off the day with some stretches even before you get out of bed. You can do stretches in the shower, walking to your car, waiting at signals, standing in line, getting up from your work station, sitting in an airport, or enduring interminable waits for your dentist or doctor. You can do a small stretch routine in the morning, on your breaks, and at lunchtime. The rest of the time, stretches can be limited to specific areas that need a respite from holding a position for a long period of time.

To give you an example of how stretching can fit into your life, I'll again refer to my own experience. When I worked at a desk, most of my work was in front of me. This meant that my shoulders were forward and my pecs contracted. It felt great to stretch back my shoulders and open my poor contracted pecs. I decided to build stretching into my daily routine. What I needed was a triggering event to help me remember to stretch. I decided that whenever I stood up for any reason, I would stretch my shoulders back. At first, I had to remember to stretch. In no time, the response was automatic. When I stood, my shoulders would squeeze back and allow my upper chest to expand. It felt good and helped me avoid the rounded shoulders so common in people who work at forward tasks all day long. (I've seen that round-shouldered appearance in people as young as 16 from hunching over books and studying without taking respites.)

The relief from stress that I felt when I stretched made me think of other places where I could insert stretching into my daily life. It had to fit easily into my life because I was busy. Without too much effort, I found many times when I could stretch.

Chapter 12: GRANDMA KNEW BEST

The next few pages contain suggested stretches for you to do. Formulate a routine for yourself. Consider the times and places that you can build in a triggering event to help you remember.

The body responds best when you stay within the rules. Take the time to read them so that your stretching is effective.

Section II: RELIEF AND PREVENTION

s-t-r-e-t-c-h-i-n-g

Rules for Stretching:

- Stretch slowly so that you can feel the limit of the stretch.
- Come out of the stretch as slowly as you went into it.
- Maintain a peaceful state of mind while stretching.
- Avoid bouncy or jerky movements when stretching.

Shoulder, Arms, and Upper Body Stretches:
(Hold the stretches for 10-15 seconds. Remember to breathe while stretching.)

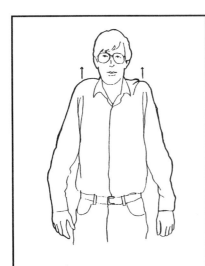

Shoulder shrugs: *Raise shoulders up towards ears. Drop shoulders.*

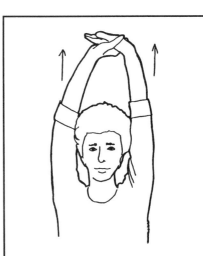

Overhead Stretch: *With palms up and arms overhead, grasp hands and pull straight up.*

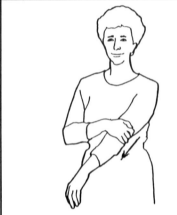

Cross Arm Stretch: *Cross arms in front. Use one hand to grasp opposite arm above elbow and pull. Change sides.*

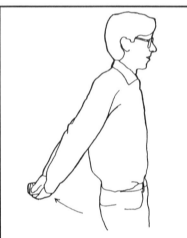

Upper Body Stretch: *Clasp hands behind back, extend and lift arms.*

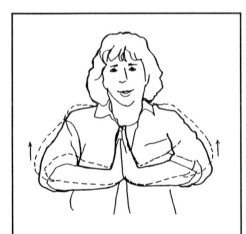

Flexor Stretch: *With palms together at chest height, slowly raise elbows.*

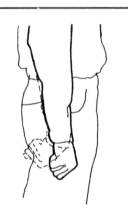

Extensor Stretch: *Place arms at sides. Make a loose fist with thumbs toward body. Bend wrists.*

Section II: RELIEF AND PREVENTION

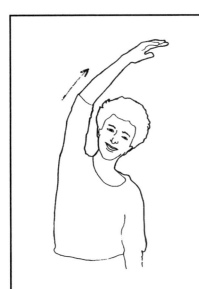

Side Bends: Raise one arm over head. Bend in the direction opposite the raised arm. Change sides.

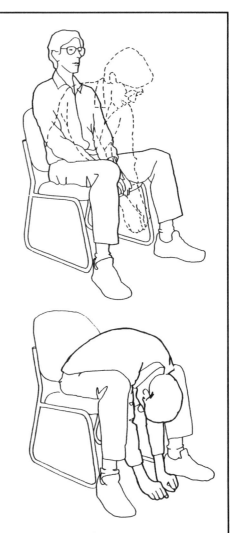

Roll Downs: Sit down with feet on floor and legs apart. Roll down slowly with arms dangling. Roll up slowly.

Chapter 12: GRANDMA KNEW BEST

Neck and Shoulder Stretches:

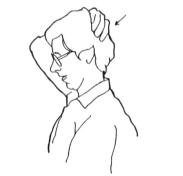

Forward Neck Stretch: *Tuck in chin. Grasp back of head. Gently push head forward.*

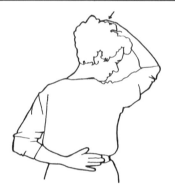

Neck/Shoulder Stretch: *Place hand in back at waist, palm out. Turn head in direction that fingers are pointing. Place free hand on crown of head and pull head down slowly. Change sides.*

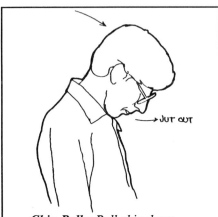

Chin Rolls: *Roll chin down until resistance. Jut out head and neck.*

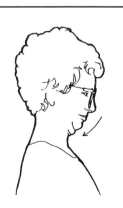

Chin Tuck Stretch: *Stretch neck upwards, then tuck in chin.*

Chapter 13:

Endurance to Spare...

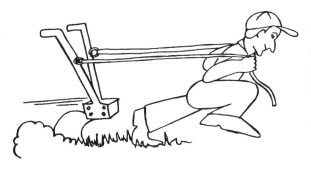

Our bodies are designed to walk long distances and to work hard when we arrive at our destination. Up until recent times, normal work and home activities provided all the exercise that people needed. Our grandparents did not need to create ways to keep their muscles strong and healthy. They tilled the soil, kneaded bread, sawed wood by hand, and walked long distances.

It is ironic that although we have many modern conveniences, we are just as busy as our grandparents were, though in a much more sedentary way. Most of us feel guilty because we are not taking care of ourselves as we know we should. We don't know how to scoop out more time for the ever growing list of "shoulds."

This problem of time constraints holds particularly true for exercise. In this chapter, after a brief explanation of the benefits of exercise to the upper body, there are a series of small exercises that will easily fit into the nooks and crannies of time that you have in a day.

Why is it necessary to exercise the upper body and arms? After all, the hands and arms and shoulders are working all day long. They certainly do not need more exercise - or so it was thought.

There is just beginning to be more emphasis on the importance of exercising the upper body and extremities. Up until recent times, the

Chapter 13: ENDURANCE TO SPARE...

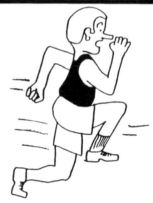

importance of exercising the lower body and legs was stressed. This is understandable. Good cardiovascular stimulation is necessary to promote a healthy heart. After all, it is a lot to ask one fist-size heart to pump blood all the way up from the feet against the force of gravity. However, there is also a need for a strong, high-endurance upper body and extremities. (Recently, I read about a marathon runner who could not carry his luggage. He had spent no time balancing the muscularization between the upper and lower halves of his body.)

In our present way of life, where repetitive motion is common, we are doing tasks that do not require physical strength, but do require physical stamina. Many of us are spending long hours doing the same thing, but without the necessary resistance to help build muscles. If we do not build stamina, then how are we to cope?

Muscles, tendons, ligaments and fascias need stretching to increase flexibility and strengthening to increase stamina. Fortunately, the upper extremities do not need heavy weights or high resistance to increase stamina. What they need is strength building over time with emphasis on light resistance and increasing repetitions. You can accomplish that during your breaks, while driving your car, staying in a hotel room, or watching television.

You can use your own body to supply resistance - as shown in the neck strengthening exercises that follow. You can also use surgical tubing or thin broad bands of elastic material - as shown in the following shoulder and upper back strengthing exercises. This is not complicated and expensive machinery. Your investment requires only one thing: The desire to feel better.

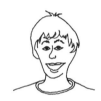

Chapter 13: ENDURANCE TO SPARE...

The Warm-up

Before exercising, it is always a good idea to warm up the body. Not only does it bring circulation into the area, it also gives the body notice to prepare to exercise.

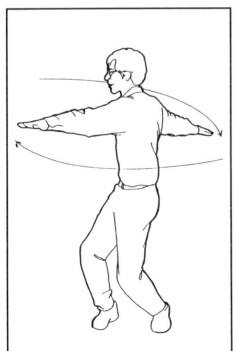

Reaching Arms: Hold arms to sides level with shoulders. Balance weight on balls of feet. Turn from side to side while bending knees.

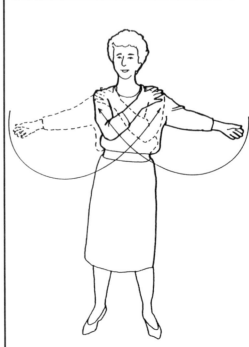

Swinging Arms: Swing arms from side to side touching opposite shoulder as you swing.

Section II: RELIEF AND PREVENTION

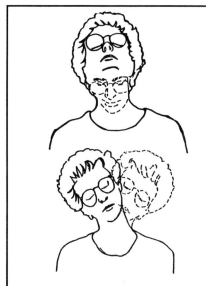

Neck Rotations: *(Caution: Be careful if you have chronic neck pain. Go slowly and STOP is there is pain.) Rotate head from front to back and from side to side.*

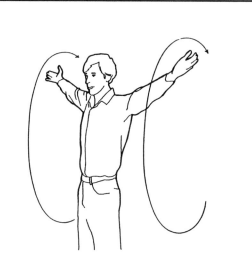

Windmills: *Using the entire arm, make circles from front to back. Repeat in opposite direction.*

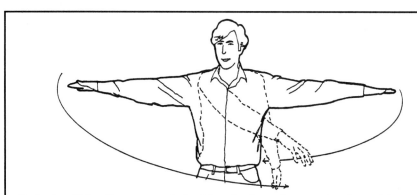

Swinging Sides: *Let arms and shoulders lead a swing, turning from side to side at the waist. Do not move hips.*

Strengthening Exercises

The material used in these illustrations is a very thin stretch band about 6 inches wide and 6 feet long. It is a fairly resistant material. You can substitute surgical tubing which comes in different diameters - the smaller the diameter, the less resistance.

If you feel pain while doing these exercises, stop immediately. If you are under a doctor's care or over 60 years of age, review these stretches with your doctor before starting.

Shoulder, Arm and Upper Body Strengtheners:
(Hold each for 5 seconds. Repeat as many as 5 times per side.)

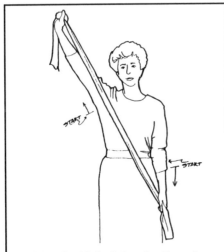

Hold band with both hands. Extend one arm down to side while pulling upward with other hand. Reverse arms.

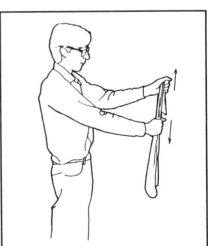

With one hand over the other, grasp band in front with both hands. Extend arms. Pull one arm up and the other arm. Reverse arms.

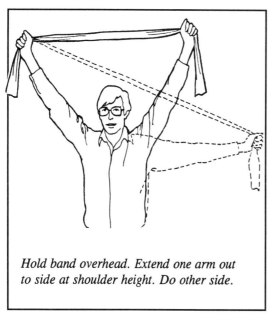

Hold band overhead. Extend one arm out to side at shoulder height. Do other side.

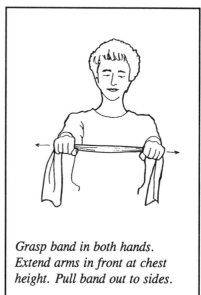

Grasp band in both hands. Extend arms in front at chest height. Pull band out to sides.

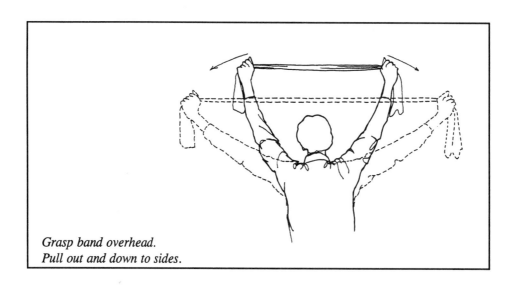

Grasp band overhead. Pull out and down to sides.

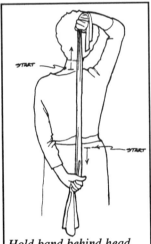

Hold band behind head. Pick up other end in back at waist. Pull in opposite directions. Change hands.

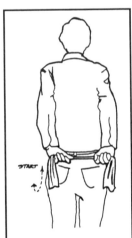

With palms up, grasp band in back of body. Extend and lift arms. Do not arch spine.

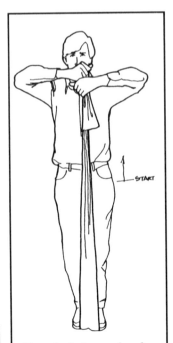

Place both feet on band. Grasp other end of band with both hands. Lift hands bending elbows out.

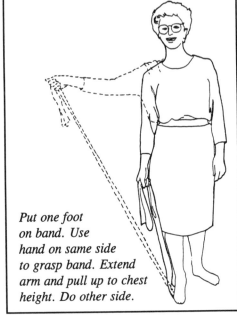

Put one foot on band. Use hand on same side to grasp band. Extend arm and pull up to chest height. Do other side.

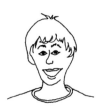

Neck Strengtheners

Neck muscles are small and do not need a lot of resistance. Use less than 50% of your strength to do these exercises.

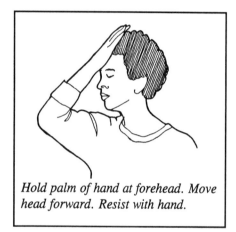

Hold palm of hand at forehead. Move head forward. Resist with hand.

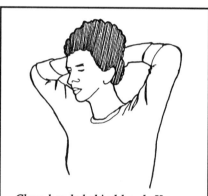

Clasp hands behind head. Keep chin level. Move head back. Resist with hands.

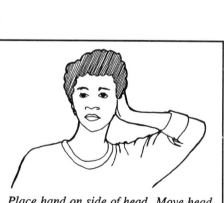

Place hand on side of head. Move head in direction of hand. Resist with hand. Do other side.

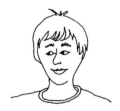

Chapter 14

LIVING AT THE TOP OF YOUR LUNGS

If you could do one small thing that would relieve your tension, calm your anger, give you energy, alleviate certain neck, shoulder and upper back pain and it took less than a minute to do, would you do it? If the answer is "yes," then read on.

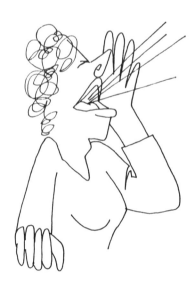

What I want to share with you is the art of breathing. I know you've been breathing all your life and think you don't need someone telling you how to do it. That's why I call what I want to share with you the "art" of breathing. Before I show you the way to do that, I would like to explain why it is important.

First of all, most of us take shallow breaths all day. We live, quite literally, at the top of our lungs. These big, wonderful organs are never fully used. Therefore, carbon dioxide which is the waste product of energy is not fully expelled and so we don't have as much room for oxygen. As a result of this shallow breathing, we do not have access to the maximum amount of energy that we need because the blood is not being sufficiently oxygenated.

This is a good place to describe what shallow breathing is. To set the stage, I'd like to give you a brief description of how the lungs breath in and out. Unlike other moving parts, the lungs have no muscles. Lung tissue is full of little air sacs (so much so that a piece of lung tissue will float in water.) In order for those little sacs to fill or empty they require the work and cooperation of surrounding muscles - namely the diaphragm and the muscles between each rib. What these muscles do is clear a space

Section II: RELIEF AND PREVENTION

for the lungs to fill with air when you take a breath. When you let it out, these muscles go back to their starting place. That is not what is happening with shallow breathing.

With shallow breathing the shoulders and neck, instead of the diaphragm, are doing the job of making a space for the lungs to expand. The little muscles which run from the upper ribs to the neck are called upon to do this exhausting work. Not only is this very hard on these small muscles but they were never designed to do this type of work. To experience this type of breathing, take a breath by moving the 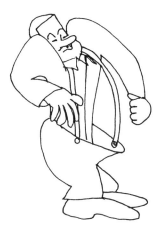 shoulders up as you inhale. This is an inefficient and ineffective way to breath. Shallow breathing leaves neck, shoulder and back muscles achy from overuse. Improper breathing could be the source of your upper body discomfort.

Another problem with shallow breathing is the expansion of tension. Remember when you were little and you played "hide -and- seek"? You would breathe very shallowly and quietly while your excitement mounted. This type of breathing produces feelings of anxiety and is associated with danger or great excitement. When you breathe that way, the body mobilizes for action. The "fight or flight" response takes hold.

Given that using the shoulders and neck to breathe is inefficient, causes muscle aches and unnecessarily mobilizes the body, wouldn't you rather learn a different way? Let's consider what is involved in a proper breath.

A properly inhaled breath focuses your attention about two inches below your belly button. In other words, as you inhale, think about sending your breath all the way down to that area of your tummy. Try it now. Take a deep breath and as you do so, concentrate on expanding that area two inches below your navel.

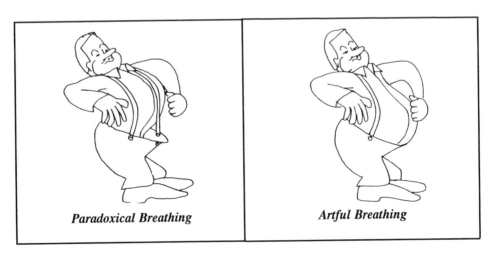

Paradoxical Breathing   *Artful Breathing*

If you are pulling in your tummy when you inhale, you are doing what is called "paradoxically breathing." This type of breathing doesn't work well because of what is happening to the diaphragm when you breath. As I mentioned earlier, the muscles around the lungs create a space for the lungs to expand. The ribs bulge out and the diaphragm drops down pushing all the organs down to create maximum capacity for the lungs. That is why the tummy swells out when you inhale and goes back in when you exhale. If you are sucking your tummy in when you inhale, then you are still breathing at the top of your lungs. Keep trying.

Section II: RELIEF AND PREVENTION

One of my clients said she was having trouble "sneaking up on her breath." Every time she thought about it, she did it right. How was she to check it? I told her not to worry. Just take a proper breath as often as possible. Place little sticky notes at home, at work and in your car with the word "BREATHE" written on them. In time, the reminders will take hold.

One last note: If you are tense, angry or anxious, breathe in making sure to expand your belly. Slow down your exhalations so that they last twice as long as your inhalations. Try it. See if you notice a shift in your sense of well-being. Try spending a minute several times a day breathing this way. Just relax and concentrate on your breathing. (These respites can also be very helpful to use before, during or after any anxiety-producing event).

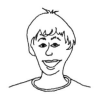

Chapter 15

EATING THE GOOD STUFF...

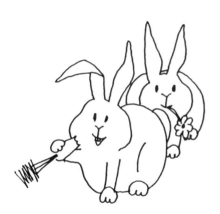

Part of asking the body to change is providing the body with the means to change. If you want to have greater stamina and more flexibility in your neck, shoulders and upper back, you have to provide the means for the body to regenerate muscle, tendon, ligament, and bone in a healthy way. One way to do that is by eating well.

To have some idea of the importance of regenerating healthy cells, I would like to repeat what I heard at a lecture by Deepak Chopra, M.D. and best selling author. Dr. Chopra told the audience that 98% of our body's atoms change once a year. He also said words to the effect that everything from skin to skeleton are changing constantly.

The question is - where does the body get the natural resources to repair and rebuild itself year after year? If your reply to the question is "from the food we eat and the fluids we drink," then you are right.

Regeneration is the key. While you rest and recuperate, the body is regenerating. It works like this: in the process of burning energy, muscles, bones, tendons, ligaments and fasciae break down their cells; during rest they regenerate new cells.

Let's look at a simple way of describing how regeneration works. Let's say that you begin a stretching program and let's say that you decide to gain more range of motion in your neck. At first, you find that you can only turn your head half the distance to your shoulder. You continue to

Section II: RELIEF AND PREVENTION

stretch throughout the day and after a while you notice that you are able to turn your head until you can look over your shoulder. What is going on? The body recognized a new need and in addition to regenerating the cells to maintain the muscles, it also generated more cells to allow your neck to turn. It was as if a message went out," We need to turn our head more, please send the nutrients we need to make this happen." The same thing occurs when you start exercising. The difference between stretching and exercising is that with exercising the muscle makes a request for nutrients in order to add bulk.

What does all this regeneration have to do with nutrition? It has just about everything to do with nutrition: If a meal consists of donuts and coffee, then that is the material the body will use to create new tissue.

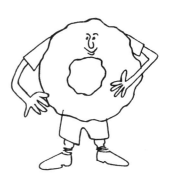

In a nutritional nutshell, the decision you make as to what you will or won't eat or drink determines what raw materials the body has for regeneration. You choose the raw material. If you eat a hot dog, the body will glean whatever cell-making nutrients it can from the hot dog. Give the body a carrot and the body will work with the nutrients from the carrot.

Eating to sustain good health, strong muscles, and high energy is confusing these days. Information changes frequently about what is good or bad for us. We are given a report that shows a new finding about a food, and a month later, we are told something entirely different. How can we know which food is right for us?

Chapter 15: EATING THE GOOD STUFF...

Whole, fresh, and uncooked food is the best. Augment fresh foods with whole grains. Add some dairy and a little fresh meat or fish (if you're so inclined.) Whatever you do, before you select food or beverage ask yourself if this is what you want to give yourself for the regeneration of YOU.

Chapter 16

IN ADDITION TO THE GOOD STUFF...

As I mentioned in the previous chapter on nutrition, if you want to feel better and heal more quickly from ailments of the shoulders, upper back and neck, you need to eat well. What if you are not sure about taking supplements? After all, there is a host of information and disagreement about whether or not there are enough vitamins and minerals in the food you eat. My thinking about dietary supplementation is that it depends. It depends on what you eat, what you assimilate, what drugs you are taking, how healthy you are and what lifestyle you have. There is no pat answer.

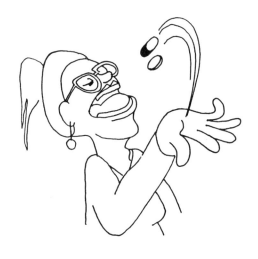

We are just as unique on the inside as we are on the outside. You may have two eyes, one nose and one mouth like everyone else, but you do not look like anyone else. The same thing is going on inside. Part of finding what is right for you involves trial and error coupled with a sense of what your body will or will not tolerate.

Sometime ago, I was talking to a woman who had wrestled with the problem of finding out what was wrong with her. She was suffering from fatigue and weakened muscles. She was tested for everything from arthritis and lupus to multiple sclerosis. Nothing was found. Finally, it was discovered that she wasn't absorbing the magnesium in the food she eats. In order to stay healthy and energetic, she has to take magnesium injections. While this is an extreme example, sometimes nutritional absorption is a problem.

Chapter 16: IN ADDITION TO THE GOOD STUFF...

There are also certain conditions or lifestyles where the amount of vitamins and minerals available in the food cannot entirely offset the need. Some of these conditions include : physical illness, pregnancy, high physical or mental stress and mental illness. Also the consumption of alcohol, birth control pills, and estrogen replacement may increase the need to supplement.

For example, vitamin B-6 has proven to be very effective in alleviating carpal tunnel syndrome <u>if the body is deficient in that particular vitamin.</u> In that case, the underlying reason for carpal tunnel syndrome is a nutritional problem.

Again, using vitamin B-6, as an example of nutritional deficiencies, what are the chances that you are getting enough vitamin B-6? The answer is, it depends. While vitamin B-6 is in most everything we eat, this vitamin is diminished or lost through canning, roasting, stewing and long storage. It would seem that if you eat lots of fresh, raw foods, you are probably getting a sufficient amount of this vitamin. However, if you have any of the conditions or lifestyles that I men- 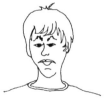 tioned in a previous paragraph or if you are taking certain drugs, supplementation might be in order.

At the end of this chapter, I have listed the supplements that professionals recommend for proper functioning and regeneration of muscles. If you think that these might be worth a try, remember to be patient. Supplements can take awhile to provide the desired results. Stay with the supplementation for at least three months.

Nutritional Supplements
to Promote Healthy Muscles and Related Tissue:

(This is for information only. Any supplementation should first be discussed with a physician.)

1. **The Electrolytes** - Minerals which are essential to prevent muscle fatigue, cramps, heat stroke and irregular heartbeats. (These are just some of the reasons for taking these minerals.)

   Potassium - You need potassium and salt on a 2:1 ratio. The American diet is just the opposite. Rather than straight table salt, try using a "Lite" salt which has potassium in it.)

   Sodium - There is usually plenty of sodium in our diet. You may not be adding salt to food cooked at home, but Americans get 75% of their salt from prepared foods.

   Chloride - Usually ingested in table salt as sodium chloride. There usually isn't any shortage of it in prepared food.

   Calcium - Much has been written about the need to build calcium strong bones and muscles. Too much phosphorus can leach calcium out of the body. Unfortunately, soda pop - especially diet soda - has a lot of phosphorus. Watch your intake of foods that are preserved with phosphates.

Magnesium - This is in short supply in a typical American diet. If you eat lots of nuts, seeds and green vegetables, you're probably getting enough. If you want to be tested, ask the doctor to do a cellular test - not a blood test.

(The other important mineral for muscles is zinc. There are supplements that have calcium, magnesium and zinc in combination.)

2. **The B-vitamins** can help reduce stress, relieve muscle cramps, and reduce edema (water retention). Since the B-Vitamins work best together, a general recommendation would be to take a Vitamin-B complex. If you have trouble digesting a Vitamin-B complex in tablet form, there are also lozenges. The potency of the lozenges should be checked to determine how much you will need to take as an appropriate trade-off for the tablets.

3. **Other Vitamins** recommended for muscle cramps or spasms are: Vitamins C, D, and E.

Chapter 17

The Water Works...

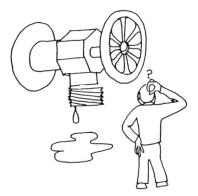

Water is so important in promoting muscle tone and reducing muscle soreness that it deserves a chapter all by itself. It is also important in preventing fatigue, headaches and joint pain. The simple change of drinking enough water every day might be enough to relieve or eliminate the pain in your shoulders, upper back and neck.

A young woman who attended my workshop had been told by her doctor that the pain in the joints of her hands and wrists was probably arthritis. That diagnosis along with some other physical problems made her decide to change her lifestyle. She began to eat better and workout. She also began to drink 2-3 quarts of water everyday. She noticed that with the increased water intake, her arthritic symptoms disappeared.

Joints need lubrication. Those bursa sacs need fluid provided by the water you drink if joints are to be maintained and tendons are to glide easily. Water is the necessary medium for carrying nutrients for regeneration and cellular repair to the muscles, tendons and fascias.

*When you do not drink sufficient water the body has to shift to a "make do" policy. The body will use whatever water it has for survival **first**.* It will store fluid and use it in a miserly way - doling out only enough to keep from totally dehydrating. The body will slow down, there will be feelings of fatigue, muscles will ache, hands and feet will swell, there may be constipation or headaches, kidney stones may form and body fat might increase.

Water is one of the least harmful and most helpful first steps that you can take toward good health. You regularly lose three quarts of water a day through sweat, urine, breathing, and other forms of elimination. You get about one quart of water from food. So, **you need at least two quarts of water to maintain**. You need more if you are under stress or heavy physical activity. Coffee should not be counted as part of your fluid intake because coffee, as well as tea and other diuretic drinks, removes approximately one-half cup of body fluid for every cup you drink.

Sports drinks are no substitute either. They are expensive and contain

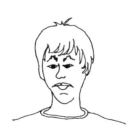 a great deal of sugar in the form of white grape juice. Undiluted juices give the body a huge sugar jolt. If you want to count juice as part of your two-quart intake, then dilute the juice by two-thirds with water. While this is not as good as pure water, at least it will cut the sugar and get more water into your body.

If you cannot stand the flavor of tap water, try steam-distilled water. It doesn't have the minerals or chlorine that might be the source of the taste you dislike. You can also put in a couple of lemon or orange slices to make the flavor more interesting. Whatever you do, don't spend time or effort on designer water.

Section II: RELIEF AND PREVENTION

Designer water, sold in cute little bottles, is very expensive and nowhere on the label does it state its purity. If you want to look fashionable, buy a bottle and drink it, save the bottle and keep refilling it with cheaper and purer distilled water. (Distilled water can be purchased by the gallon for under $1.00. I have bought it on sale for as little as $.30 a gallon.)

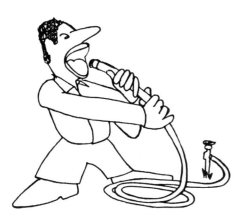

If the idea of drinking a large volume of water each day seems difficult, my suggestion is that you invest in a couple of those quart-size sip bottles. Keep one on your desk and the other near your easy chair or in your car. I know how hard it is to look at a whole quart of water and imagine getting through it. There is something about having a handy sip bottle that makes a person reach over and drink. It is remarkable what an easy way that is to drink the water you need.

If your reason for not drinking a lot of water is that you will have to go to the bathroom frequently then you need to know that as your body adjusts to the additional fluid, you will not need to urinate quite so often. Besides, those bathroom trips will not only give you a rest from repetitive motion, but also give you an opportunity to stretch, breath, or do some other activity that will help you. What a good deal!

One last thing: don't wait for feelings of thirst. Adults cannot rely on the thirst signal. For one thing, the less water you drink, the less you crave. For another, signals for thirst get confused with signals of hunger. You might try drinking a glass of water and waiting 20 minutes to see if you're still hungry. It could have been thirst and not hunger that needed satisfying.

Give water a try. What have you got to lose except your tiredness, your muscle soreness and the pain in your joints?

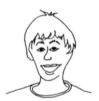

Chapter 18

Rubbing Away the Owies...

The first thing we do whenever we bang into the furniture is to rub the offended part of our body. (Maybe it is the second thing we do right on the heels of saying something extremely rude to the offending furniture.) Even toddlers will rub a spot that has an owie. It seems instinctive to massage a hurt.

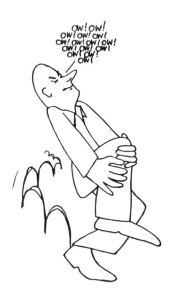

One of the effects of rubbing an area is to increase the circulation in that area. Perhaps instinct guides us, because massaging the owie increases the nutrient-rich blood supply and hastens healing. Another benefit of rubbing is to help relax the injured area. It would seem that self-massage is a natural reaction to certain types of injuries.

Unfortunately, the wonderful rubbing instinct only seems to kick in when the pain is sudden and overwhelming. In the day to day world of wear and tear, we often try to ride out the tension and pain that we feel.

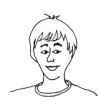

In my own professional experience, I have observed that the process of massage not only brings the nutrients but also the attention of the mind and body to the injured area. As I mentioned in an earlier chapter, cumulative trauma sneaks up on you. The twinge, the tingling, the little spasm, and the muscle tension can all be overlooked until the pain is great enough or the discomfort lasts long enough to focus your attention and generate action on your part. Before the problem reaches such levels of pain, you can use massage to help the area.

In this chapter, I will give you various massage techniques that you can use to help yourself. There is one area that you probably cannot reach - that spot right between the shoulder blades. For those unreachable areas, you can buy a special wooden dowel which you can place on the floor and lie on to relieve the tension spots. The dowel is available at health stores, massage supply stores or through catalogs.

For the rest of your upper body and extremities, try the massage routine that follows. It will do you a world of good.

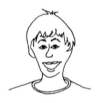

Section II: RELIEF AND PREVENTION

Self-Massage for Head, Neck, and Shoulders

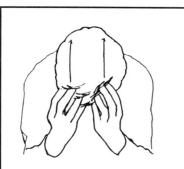

Place both hands on the forehead. Massage back and down to nape of neck. Be sure to move scalp.

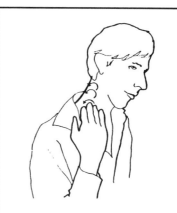

Starting at collarbone, use one hand to massage side of neck with small circles up to nape of neck. Do other side.

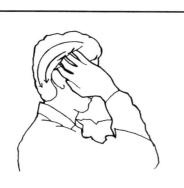

Use both hands. Start at temples, massage back over ears to nape of neck. Be sure to move scalp.

Chapter 18: RUBBING AWAY THE OWIES...

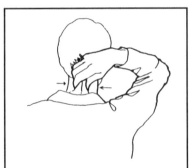

Starting at base of neck at spine, use hand to squeeze neck up to scalp. Change hands and repeat.

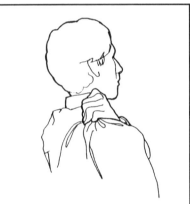

Use hand to squeeze opposite shoulder. Start at base of neck. Continue down to arm. Do both inside and outside of arm. Do other side.

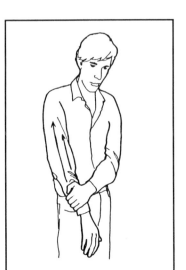

Use long strokes up arm to shoulder. Do other shoulder and arm.

Chapter 19

Sleeping Through It...

How many times have you awakened in the morning with a stiff neck or shoulder pain? You take inventory of your night's sleep and can't think of a reason. You will probably conclude that you "slept funny" and you are probably right.

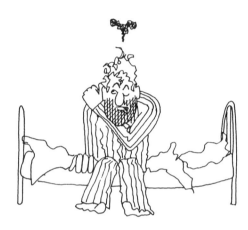

There are several causes for waking up with neck pain. The first one could be the way you sleep. If you like to sleep on your tummy, then you are forcing your head to one side which keeps the neck turned during the night.

People who sleep on their tummies often sleep with their arms extended over their heads. This sleep position can cause pain in the shoulders. The extension of the arms over the head cuts off blood and nerve circulation into the hands. You can wake up with the same sensations as someone with carpal tunnel syndrome. Another very good reason for not sleeping on your tummy is that it forces the lower back into an extreme curve and it puts a great deal of pressure on that part of the spine.

What can you do to change the tendency to sleep on your tummy? Get some bolsters or pillows and place them beside you in bed. If you roll on them, you'll probably stop midway which will leave you lying on your side. You can also try a body pillow. Some people find that a cervical roll or a pillow with a slight depression for their head discourages sleeping on their tummies. Whatever you do, stay with it. There is much to gain by breaking the habit of sleeping face down.

Another reason for morning pain may have to do with the headrest that you use. As I indicated in an earlier chapter, if you like to watch TV or read while lying on your back or side with your head elevated, then you are a candidate for neck pain. The same applies to sleeping on a poorly designed pillow. (Watch those sofa arms.)

A too plump pillow can raise the head and cause the spine to bend at the neck, thereby straining the muscles and ligaments. A pillow which is too low can drop the head back also causing neck strain. What can be done to find a just-right pillow?

There are a wide variety of shapes and sizes of headrests. You will need to try different ones. Make sure that you can get an exchange or refund. Try the headrest on you own bed. You can't judge it by trying it out on a bed in the store because the mattress may be firmer or softer than yours. For proper support, the headrest needs to support your head and neck but not extend down to the shoulders. (**Shoulders should never rest on the pillow.**)

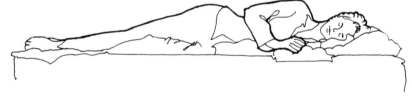

Use your x-ray vision to make sure that your spine is aligned from the base of your neck to the end of your tailbone. If you can feel that your neck is not aligned in every direction, look for another headrest.

Section II: RELIEF AND PREVENTION

Check the condition of your pillow or headrest every 3 months. It could have become misshapen or flattened. If so, it is time to replace it.

If you sleep sitting up, find a comfortable head and neck support that won't allow your head to drop or turn to one side. (The same rule applies if you like to sleep on your back.) Use an inflatable neck and headrest when you are traveling in a car or plane to hold your head straight.

One final thought: If you tend to sleep on your side but your shoulder is bothering you and you can't get comfortable, put a pillow next to your chest and rest your upper arm on it. This will keep your shoulder from rolling forward and help you maintain a more neutral position for the shoulder.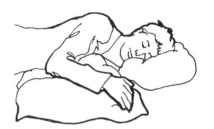

Chapter 20

The Tension Troublespots...

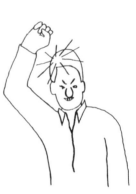

At the end of a highly productive but stressful day, it's no fun to go home with a raging tension headache, eyestrain, or TMJ symptoms. In this chapter, we will look at the cause of each of these culprits and what you can do about them.

Tension headaches:

Tension headaches are usually the result of stressed neck ligaments Go back to Chapter 10 where I explain about positioning your body. Make your environment and posture fit the four rules of positioning that the body likes best as listed in that chapter.

Here are some other ideas to help you rid yourself of tension headaches:

Focus on the pain.
A natural response to pain is to tense. However, tension further increases the pain. In order to relax, try the following relaxation technique: Take several deep breaths as described in Chapter 14. Close your eyes and ask yourself the following questions while doing the breathing: Where is the pain? What is the color of the pain? What is the shape of the pain? How much water would it hold?

Use your hands to relieve the pain.
Massage around your ears. Then gently pull your ears down and hold for 5 seconds. Then pull up for 5 seconds and then pull back for 5 seconds. Now massage the scalp making sure to actually *move* the scalp as you do it. Then reach up to the top of your head and grasp the hair very close to the roots. Lightly pull on your hair towards your face with just enough

pressure so that you can feel the scalp tightening. Hold for 5 seconds. Continue holding the hair and pull towards the back of the head. Do the same thing to the hair on the sides of your head. Be sure to pull in all directions. That will stretch the muscles and fascias of the head and neck. (This exercise is very helpful if you tend to squint or frown.)

Use acupressure to help.
Apply a comfortable pressure to each spot. Keep finger pressure steady and take 3 deep breaths at each acupressure point:

(1) Pinch the webbing between the thumb and index finger

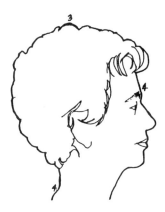

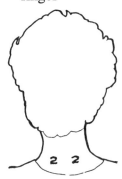

(2) press in on both sides of the spine just at the base of the neck

(3) press in at the very crown of the head; (4) simultaneously press the middle of the forehead and base of the neck at the middle of the spine.

Chapter 20: THE TENSION TROUBLESPOTS...

Take away pain with hydrotherapy.
Ice on the back of the neck can often relieve a tension headache. If you don't have an ice bag, you can use a bag of frozen peas or corn to lie on. Leave on for about 10 minutes. Taking a warm bath helps relieve headaches. (You can put herbs such as hops, valerian root or skullcap in the bath to help enhance relaxation.)

Eyestrain:

Eyestrain is one of the workplace problems the National Institute of Occupational Safety and Health (NIOSH) has considerably studied. Chronic eyestrain can lead to tension in the neck, shoulders and upper back. Computer monitors are not the only source of the problem. Anything that has to do with continuous, close vision can lead to eyestrain, including TV watching, reading and hobbies involving close work.

In addition to making postural corrections, here are suggestions for eliminating or reducing eyestrain:

Extend the distance to the object.
Most computer screens are located too close to the eyes. Move the screen at least 22 inches from your eyes. Measure the distance from the TV screen, also.

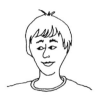

Correct any glare.
Primary and secondary glare is a big culprit in eyestrain. Primary glare

refers to natural or artificial light directly hitting the eyes. Invest in blinds for the windows so that light can be directed away from your eyes. If you are doing close work, turn down the overhead light and concentrate on using task lights. (I often suggest desk lamps for paper work. Also, there are small clamp-on tensor lamps to put on document holders for transcribing.)

Secondary glare is the light that bounces off of an object and into your eyes. For example, I corrected a receptionist station where the overhead lights bounced off of the plastic mat on top of the desk. If you use a computer screen, turn it off and note where light is reflecting. Get a good screen filter or hood to block the light, decrease the contrast, or change the work station to a different location.

Exercise the eyes.
Every 10 minutes, look up and observe something at a distance. Every hour, close your eyes and rest them for a few minutes.

Apply acupressure to tired eyes.
Use the same techniques as described for headaches to the following areas:

(1) Press your index fingers at the cheek ridge just below the middle of the eye; (2) press the indentation just at the outside corner of the eye; (3) press on both sides of the root of the bridge of the nose.

Other help for tired eyes:

Dampen cotton pads with witch hazel and place over eyelids for 10 minutes while you lie down and relax. (Keep witch hazel in refrigerator. The cold will help reduce any swelling around the eyes.) If you don't have witch hazel, you can use moistened tea bags.

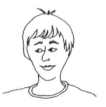

TMJ Symptoms:

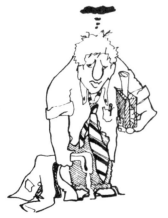

The last tension troublemaker in this chapter is TMJ problems. TMJ is the brief name given to a multisyllable medical word to describe the jaw joint. Symptoms of TMJ include jaw clicking, popping, grating or inability to fully open your mouth. Assuming that your teeth are aligned and you haven't suffered an injury to your jaw, the reason for TMJ might be tension.

Grinding or clenching your teeth either while awake or asleep could be the cause of TMJ. You may want to get a device from the dentist to keep you from grinding your teeth at night. Poor posture and body alignment could also be responsible. You need to line up your body in accordance with the four postural rules described in Chapter 10. Also, pay particular attention to activities which cause you to have your head tilted back.

Section II: RELIEF AND PREVENTION

Here are ideas for you to help alleviate the symptoms of TMJ:

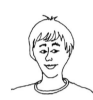

Make changes in your daily activities.
The phone receiver can apply continuous pressure on your jaw, especially near your ear. Chewing gum can also aggravate TMJ.

Massage the area
Massage and pull the scalp and ears as recommended for headaches. Massage the jaws, too.

Heat and stretch the jaw.
Take a steamy hot towel and place across chin to reach on both sides of jaw. Hold for about 15 minutes.

When you have finished heating the jaw with the hot towel do the following exercises while looking in the mirror:

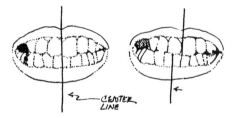

Slowly and *gently* move the lower jaw so that you are over one tooth from center. Do this 5 times in each direction. Next, *slowly* jut jaw forward until upper and lower teeth meet. Relax and do again. Repeat 5 times.

Use isometric exercises to strengthen jaw muscle.
(You do not need to use more than light resistance to do these.)

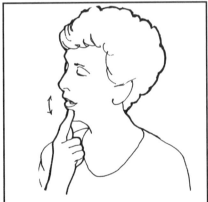

Relax jaw. Place a finger in indentation above chin. Open jaw against light resistance from finger.

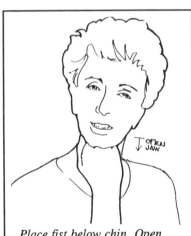

Place fist below chin. Open jaw against light resistance from fist.

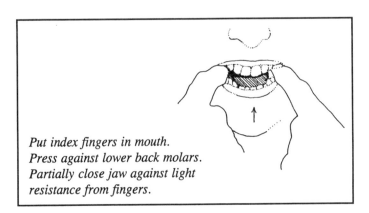

Put index fingers in mouth. Press against lower back molars. Partially close jaw against light resistance from fingers.

Chapter 21

A Few Last Thoughts...

One of the easiest things to do is to override the signals from your body - especially if it has to do with wear and tear. Perhaps you were raised to believe that working was about enduring. Or maybe you feel that the greatest priority is getting the task done - no matter what. Those beliefs can quickly lead to a painful shoulder, a crick in the neck, or an ache in the middle of your back that will not let up.

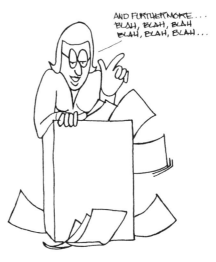

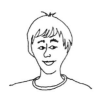
Good health and a sense of well-being are good reasons to vary your routine and give your body and mind a break. Besides, information gathered on productive work habits shows that **non-stop working isn't very effective.** You actually will finish your task with more ease and more efficiency if you vary what you are doing.

A good example of task variation is a personal one. I had set aside one weekend to sand and paint the trim on the house. I don't particularly like to sand or paint so I wanted to finish as quickly as possible. The garage door proved to be more work than I had anticipated. Part of me wanted to endure and get the job done. Fortunately, a wiser part of me prevailed. I knew that I needed a break often because I was using continuous force against the garage door and the sander was vibrating my hand and arm. (As stated earlier in this book, repetitions with force and vibration can quickly lead to problems.) What I needed to do was

Chapter 21: A FEW LAST THOUGHTS...

take frequent breaks from the force and vibration. So, I brought out a clock and set it for 15 minutes. I got the job done... 15 minutes on and 10 minutes off. I finished the job in the time I had allotted, but without feeling aggravated and without injuring myself.

When you are preparing to do anything, think about the best way to accomplish it physically. As I said in an earlier chapter, if you find that your body is resisting, do not force it. Act kindly. Figure out what you need to change so that the body can do the work more easily. Every Monday, I get phone calls from clients who have spent the weekend doing too much and now have sore backs, pulled muscles, and strained tendons or ligaments. Learn what the capacity of your body and mind is, and stay within those markers.

If you are getting bored or your body is getting tired of the position, do something else. Get a drink of water. Do a little stretching. Shake out your arms. Look off into the horizon. Do a different chore. Whatever you do, vary your day, your task, and your activity.

Before you start a task, ask yourself how you can make it more fun and less wearing.

Another way to help yourself is to eat consciously and drink plenty of water. It takes just as much time to get a hot dog and a coke at a fast food restaurant as it does to throw some fruits and veggies into a lunch sack. Then, when it is time to eat, instead of driving off to the nearest convenience store or fast food joint, you can use the time to eat and take a walk. (That way, you don't have to get up early to exercise.) If you use your lunchtime to go shopping, pay bills, or do your banking, could you possibly walk three times a week and do errands on the other two days? This is what I mean by fitting healthier changes into your day.

Throughout this book, I have made suggestions for caring for yourself within your regular daily schedule. Try to live a life with fewer of the dreaded "shoulds." Do what you can. Add little changes here or there. (There is a chart in the back of this book to help you work out a plan.) Above all, treat your body as an equal partner on this journey.

Appendix A

Home Treatment of Injuries...

___

Home Treatment of Tendinitis, Sprains and other Soft Tissue Injuries

Before you start treating yourself or anyone else, be sure to talk with your physician. He or she may want to examine the injury first. If you suspect that the bone is broken or if the trauma is serious, you need to immobilize the area and see your doctor immediately.

The techniques described below are to be used only in cases of a minor muscle pull, sprain, tendinitis, whiplash, or bursitis as determined by your physician.

For the first 48 hours after the injury, use the **RICE** formula:

R is for Resting the area of injury. At the very least, rest means to take it easy. However, if there is a lot of pain, then it might be better to completely immobilize the area.

I is for Icing the area. Place an ice bag (or ice cubes in a plastic bag and wrapped in a towel) on the area. Leave on for 10 minutes. Do this every hour. You can also do an ice massage. Fill a paper or styrofoam cup with water and place in freezer. When the water is frozen, tear around the edge of the cup and massage the injured area with the ice. (This is an easy way to ice a joint.)

C is for Compression. Use an elastic bandage to compress the injury. Remember, this is not a tourniquet so keep the compression firm, but not tight. You want to keep swelling down without cutting off the circulation.

E is for Elevating. Try to keep the injured area elevated so that fluids cannot pool and cause swelling.

Appendix A: HOME TREATMENT OF INJURIES...

After 48 hours, you can do light massage and gentle stretching if you can do so without pain. This is a good time to begin the alternating hot and cold treatment. Start and end with heat - preferably moist heat such as a shower, wet towel or a tub soak. Alternate 10 minutes of heat with 5 minutes of cold.

After massaging the area, see if you can find any particularly sore spots. Apply light pressure to the spot while closing your eyes, taking 3 deep breaths (as described in Chapter 14), relaxing and focusing on the place where you are applying pressure.

Appendix B

Your Plan of Action

On this page and the next are examples of charts that you can use to start taking action for yourself. After you have completed the chart, make up reminders using sticky paper or plain paper and tape. Place the note to yourself in an appropriate place... the car dash, your computer screen, or your locker.

This plan belongs to:

My Plan of Action

BY: (date to finish)	I WILL HAVE MADE THE FOLLOWING CHANGES: (Ergonomic changes to work station, home, car, hobby area, etc.)	Completed (date)	Comments:

BEST TIMES TO TAKE CARE OF MYSELF

ACTIVITY and COMMENT	In the morning	On the morning commute	During the day	On my breaks	At lunchtime	On the evening commute	At home	At hobbies or sports
Stress Relief								
Mini-vacations								
Ergonomics								
Stretching								
Strengthening								
Self Massage								
Acupressure								
Nutrition								
Supplementation (Nutritional)								
Isometrics								
Daily Activity								
Other								

Glossary

acute: having a short and rather severe course

carpal tunnel: wrist tunnel which is the passageway for the median nerve and the tendons that flex your fingers

chronic: long duration or frequent recurrence

compression: squeezing together; action exerted upon a body which tends to increase its density

congenital: existing at birth

contract (muscle): to draw shorter and broader

cumulative trauma disorder: type of injury usually developing gradually as a result of repeated microtrauma

deviation: a turning away or aside from the normal point

diagnosis: identifying a disease by its signs or symptoms

expand (muscle): to increase in size; to draw longer and narrower

flexibility: readily bent without breaking

ganglionic cysts: a tendon sheath disorder in which the sheath swells and causes a bump under the skin, usually at the wrist

golfer's elbow: (medial epicondylitis) irritation of the tendons at their attachment on the inside of the elbow

health: the condition of being sound in body, mind, and soul; freedom from physical disease or pain

inflammation: a local response to an injury of swelling, redness, pain and heat

kyphosis: abnormal outward curvature of the spine

ligament: a tough band of tissue connecting bone to bone

lordosis: abnormal inward curvature of the spine

massage: systematic therapeutic friction, stroking or kneading of the body

minerals: inorganic compounds or elements

mobility: capacity to move or be moved

muscles: tissues that are capable of contracting and function to produce motion

GLOSSARY

muscle fiber: the tissue that contracts when stimulated

nerves: tissue that when stimulated carried impulse to act

nutrition: the process by which food is taken in and processed

nutritional supplements: something that complements or makes an addition to food

pinched nerve: a nerve which is being squeezed or compressed painfully

predisposing conditions: to be susceptible or inclined to certain disease or disorder

prevention: to take action in advance against something happening

referred pain: pain felt in a part of the body at some distance for the source of the pain

regenerate: to form or create again

relief: removal or lessening of pain

repetitive motion injury: the pain or discomfort experienced when repeated movement thickens the tendons' lubricating membranes thereby squeezing nerves against bone and ligament

resistance (muscle): to exert force in opposition to the muscle

rigidity: lacking flexibility; stiff, hard

rotator cuff: name given to four reinforcing muscles that extend from the scapula (shoulder) to the humerus (upper arm)

rotator cuff tendinitis: common shoulder disorder also known as supraspinatus tendinitis, subdeltoid bursitis, subacromial bursitis, and partial tear of the cuff

scoliosis: curvature of the spine from side to side

signs: objective evidence of disease

spasms: involuntary and abnormal muscle contraction

stamina: staying power, endurance

strength (training): power to resist force

stress: bodily or mental tension that maybe a factor in disease

GLOSSARY

stretching: extending the body or limbs

symptoms: subjective evidence of disease

syndromes: a group of signs and symptoms that occur together and are characteristic of a certain disease or disorder

systemic: affecting the whole body

tendons: the band or cord that unites a muscle to bone and transmits the force which the muscle exerts

tendinitis: inflammation of the tendon due to overuse or misuse; commonly use to describe any inflammation of the elbow and surrounding area

tennis elbow (lateral epicondylitis): muscles that control the movement of the finger and hand which attach at the elbow are irritated from overuse and misuse

thoracic outlet syndrome: a condition in which poor neck and shoulder posture or a cervical rib put pressure on the nerve root which passes from the neck to the arm.

twinges: a sudden, sharp local pain

variety: changing from time to time

vitamin: organic substances that are essential to the body in small quantities and act in the regulation of metabolic processes

water: the liquid that is a major part of all living matter

Index

INDEX

INDEX

Biographical Sketch

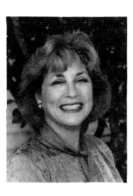

Rosemarie Atencio is a consultant, lecturer and author in the areas of health, stress management and ergonomics.

In 1987 after making a career transition, Rosemarie completed her internship in San Diego and received her certification as a health practitioner. Her specialized studies included kinesiology, psychology, nutrition, ergonomics, exercise, anatomy, and physiology.

Upon completion of her education, she returned to Eugene, Oregon, to establish a private health practice. Beginning in 1991, she extended her workshops and consulting to businesses and trade/professional organizations.

Rosemarie holds a college teaching credential and has served on the advisory board of two colleges. She has presented programs at local, state, and regional levels for professional organizations, and has been interviewed and featured nationwide on radio and television on the subject of repetitive motion injuries and ergonomics.

Rosemarie has two books in print: <u>Carpal Tunnel Syndrome: How to Relieve and Prevent Wrist "Burnout"!</u> and <u>Free Yourself from Pain in the Shoulders, Upper Back and Neck.</u>

SPECIAL REPORTS FOR YOU...

Do you want to feel better right away? Then don't wait until you are diagnosed with tendinitis, thoracic outlet syndrome, carpal tunnel syndrome or any of the other wear and tear disorders. Be proactive. You don't have to "put up" with muscle pain anymore. The following reports can guide you to a pain-free life:

SR101: How to Make Your Work Area Work FOR you Instead of AGAINST You. You will learn how to adjust your work station to fit you instead of fitting yourself to the work station. These changes alone can save you unnecessary stress and pain.

SR102: At Last! Self-Massages for the Upper Body and Upper Extremities. (You Can Use this Routine on Significant Others, Too) Get rid of inflammation, water retention and slow circulation. These techniques will make you feel like a million!

SR103: How to Avoid or Relieve Carpal Tunnel Syndrome and Other Repetitive Motion Injuries When Using a Keyboard, Mouse or Stylus. You do not need to suffer pain because you use a computer... not after you read this report. This report is full of easy techniques you can use to get relief.

SR104: How to Get Stress Relief from Artful Breathing and Acupressure Points: Acupressure is the same as acupuncture - without the needles - just thumb pressure. When you combine it with artful breathing, you get immediate stress relief.

SR105: How to Maximize Your Nutrition to Relieve Repetitive Strain and Keep Your Muscles Healthy. The old expression, "you are what you eat" has never been more true. Learn about the foods that will give you strong muscles, healthy bones and high energy.

SR106: Herbs that Help You Get Relief from Repetitive Strain Injuries. In your cupboard or at your local nutrition store are hundreds of helpful herbs. You can get relief from bruises, muscle aches, and joint discomfort.

More Special Reports and order form on the next page...

SR107: How Hydrotherapy Can Relieve & Prevent Repetitive Motion Injuries. Water in its many forms - ice, steam, hot or cold liquid, has long been recognized in relief and prevention of strains and muscle pain. There is no more plentiful and easy-to-use ingredient for a pain-free life.

SR108: How to Stand, Sit, or Lift Comfortably. To avoid the blues of aching backs, pulled muscles and strained necks, you need this handy report. You'll learn how to avoid standing, sitting and lifting in ways that leave you aching.

SR109: How to Get a Good Night's Rest and Wake Up Feeling Good. You don't need to wake up anymore because your fingers are tingling. Nor do you need to wake up in the morning with your neck and shoulders aching.

SR110A-D: How to Prevent Carpal Tunnel Syndrome and Upper Back Problems for the: SR110A: Gardener, SR110B:Musician, SR110C:Artist, SR110D: Professional Driver. (Order by number plus the letter)Each report detail techniques for prevention/relief of repetitive motion injuries and how you can apply the techniques specifically to your profession or hobby.

SR111: How to Prevent or Get Relief from Tension Headaches and Eyestrain. Headaches and eyestrain need not bother you anymore. In this easy-to-read report, you learn the tricks for eliminating the problems.

SR112: How to Arrive at Your Destination Feeling Good without Stiffness or Muscle Tension. Whether you are traveling by car, train, plane or bus, you can arrive at your destination feeling relaxed and free of muscle tightness.

SR113: How to Enjoy Sports and Avoid Repetitive Motion Injuries. Tennis, bicycling, and golf are some of the sports that can raise havoc with the upper body and extremities. It doesn't have to be that way and you will find out why in this report.

Each report is $6.00. You can SAVE $3.00 by ordering three (3) for $15.00!

You can order Special Reports on your Mastercard or Visa or send a check to: HWD Publishing, PO Box 220, Veneta, OR 97487

❑ Yes! Send me the following report numbers: ─────────────
─────────────────────────────────────

Visa/Mastercard # _____
Expiration Date: _____ Name on Card: _____
Mail to: (Name/Address) _____

(Please include $.75 for each report for postage and shipping)

From HWD Publishing...

Book:

CARPAL TUNNEL SYNDROME: How to Relieve and Prevent Wrist "Burnout"

Designed with you in mind. Whatever your occupation, profession or job, this book is crammed with good ideas for the care of your hands, wrist and forearms. ISBN 0-9637360-1-9 $13.95 plus shipping/ handling

Video Tape:

CARPAL TUNNEL SYNDROME: Relief & Prevention, The Short Course

Practical, easy-to-follow demonstrations of stretching, strengthening, massage, and correct wrist movements. 20 min. VHS, ISBN 0-9637360-3-5 $21.95 plus shipping/handling

---

Book:

SHOULDERS, UPPER BACK & NECK: Free Yourself from PAIN

You don't have to be in pain anymore. This easy-to-read book (over 100 illustrations) can help you get rid of pain immediately.   ISBN 0-9637360-9-4 $17.95 plus shipping/handling

Video Tape:

SHOULDERS, UPPER BACK & NECK: Relief & Prevention: The Short Course.

Don't let upper body pain get you down. Learn the stretching, strengthening, self-massage, and tension terminator techniques that will end the pain. 20 min. VHS, ISBN 0-9637360-5-1 $21.95 plus shipping/handling

---

Posters:

Laminated 8 ½ x 11 poster for office, home or anywhere else you need to have a reminder. $4.95 each plus s/h - unless stated otherwise

Hand and Wrist Stretching/Strengthening (with set of 3 exercise balls - $11.95)

Shoulders, Upper Back & Neck Exercises (with 6 foot latex exercise tube - $11.95)

Shoulders, Upper Back & Neck Stretches

Tension Terminators (How-to body movements w/illustrations to relieve tension)

Special Offer: Buy the Book and the Video at the same time and get a black and white laminated poster **FREE!... a SAVINGS OF $4.95!**

After you've read the book, give us your opinion and we'll send you a **FREE** 1-year's subscription to the *NoStress Newsletter*.
(see next page for details)

Fill out this portion to order and to receive your FREE subscription:

Company: _____

Your Name: _____ Title: _____

Address: _____

City: _____ State: _____ Zip: _____

I found the book to be: _____

_____

_____

May we quote you? ❑ Yes   ❑ No

Order Form

Item	Price	Quantity	Total
Carpal Tunnel Syndrome:			
Book , Tape AND FREE Poster	$35.90		
Book	$13.95		
Video Tape	$21.95		
Shoulders, Upper Back & Neck:			
Book, Tape AND FREE Poster	$39.90		
Book	$17.95		
Video Tape	$21.95		
Posters:			
Hand and Wrist Exercises	$ 4.95		
(With set of 3 balls)	$11.95		
Shoulders etc - Exercises	$ 4.95		
(With 6ft latex tube)	$11.95		
Shoulders etc - Stretching	$ 4.95		
Tension Terminators	$ 4.95		

For VISA/Mastercard, call 1+800-935-7323 .

Send check or money order (do not send cash) to: HWD Publishing, PO Box 220, Veneta, OR 97487.

For quantity discounts, call (503) 935-1608

Subtotal: $ _____

Shipping/Handling: $3.50 _____

Total Enclosed: $ _____

Allow 2-3 weeks for delivery

Satisfaction guaranteed or your money back